Prescription TV

# Prescription TV

## THERAPEUTIC DISCOURSE IN THE HOSPITAL AND AT HOME

Joy V. Fuqua

Duke University Press   Durham & London   2012

© 2012 Duke University Press
All rights reserved
Printed in the United States of America
on acid-free paper ∞
Designed by Katy Clove
Typeset in Warnock Pro by Keystone Typesetting, Inc.
Library of Congress Cataloging-in-Publication Data
appear on the last printed page of this book.

*For my parents*

# Contents

**ACKNOWLEDGMENTS** ix

**INTRODUCTION** Television, Hospital, Home 1

1. Convalescent Companions:
   Hospital Entertainment before Television 23

2. Television Goes to the Modern Hospital 49

3. Positioning the Patient:
   The Spatial Therapeutics of Hospital Television 71

4. Television in and out of the Hospital:
   Broadcasting Directly to the Consumer-Patient 93

5. Mediated Agency: Consumer-Patients and
   Pfizer's Viagra Commercials 115

**CONCLUSION** Our Bodies, Our (TV) Selves 141

**NOTES** 155

**SELECTED BIBLIOGRAPHY** 187

**INDEX** 197

**Acknowledgments**

Book acknowledgments sometimes start with an explanation of the beginning of, or inspiration behind, the author's project. Following that generic format, I would have to say that I owe my book's origin, as well as its inspiration, to different contexts. The first context extends all the way back to my childhood when my parents, in an effort to improve my scholastic math performance, forbade me to watch television. Eventually, my parents understood that there was no direct, cause-effect relationship between television viewing and second-grade math scores. If it is the case that one is inevitably drawn to the thing that one cannot have, then perhaps it is because I was denied television that I became increasingly curious about it.

The second context to which this book owes its upbringing is explicitly tied to browsing library open stacks. If it were not for the browsing possibilities provided by the open stacks policies at several university libraries, this book might never have been written. It was literally by chance and curiosity that I came on the topic of television in hospitals. For allowing access to books, journals, and magazines, I am truly grateful to the librarians, archivists, library administrators, and photocopy machine technicians at numerous libraries across the United States.

I owe an intellectual debt to my teachers, including Danae Clark, Eric O. Clarke, Ann Cvetkovich, Jane Feuer, Barbara Harlow, Marcia Landy, Dana Polan, and Janet Staiger. Each of these scholars taught me that there is such a thing as interdisciplinary research, and that popular culture is worth studying, theorizing, and writing about. Most of all, they encouraged intellectual adventure and taught me how to convey that first, necessary quality to my students.

As is the case with most books, many minds, hands, and hearts have influenced its shape, from mentors, colleagues, editors, readers, archivists, students, and friends to people sitting next to me on the subway. This project, as it grew and developed, has received support from different institutions. Tulane University provided a junior faculty summer research grant during the book's early stages. Additionally, I was awarded a J. William Fulbright Scholar Grant (2005) that allowed me to teach at the City University of Hong Kong and to further develop the project. While in Hong Kong, a number of colleagues and friends extended their hospitality and intellectual support to me. I would like to give my special thanks to Catherine Cloran, John Erni, C. C. Lee, Gina Marchetti, Anissa Tung, and the administration, faculty, and students at City University of Hong Kong.

Research librarians, archivists, and support staff have been vital to the completion of this project. I thank the following Tulane University libraries: Howard-Tilton Memorial Library; Architecture Library; Lillian A. and Robert L. Turchin Library; and Rudolph Matas Library of the Health Sciences. Additional research was conducted at Louisiana State University Health Sciences Center Library; the American Institute of the History of Pharmacy at the University of Wisconsin, Madison; and the National Library of Medicine. I received personalized research and archival assistance from several librarians and researchers, such as Beatrice Calvert, Rosemary Hanes (Library of Congress), Dr. Gregory J. Higby (director of the American Institute of the History of Pharmacy), Mary Holt, Allyson Mackay, Polly Thistlethwaite (City University of New York, Graduate Center), and Susan Tucker.

Professional conferences have also been invaluable platforms for the elaboration of the book's chapters. Console-ing Passions was the conference at which I first gave the preliminary conference paper that shaped the book. I want to acknowledge the feminist television and media scholars of Console-ing Passions for being not only my mentors, but also my colleagues and my friends. For providing supportive mentoring through the conferences, and beyond them, I especially thank Jackie Cook, Julie D'Acci, Mary Desjardins, Anna Everett, Jane Feuer, Mary Beth Haralovich, Heather Hendershot, Michele Hilmes, Carol Stabile, and Mimi White. Other feminist television scholarship has been very influential, including the work of Lynn Spigel and Anna McCarthy. The Society for Cinema and Media Studies (SCMS) has provided another important forum for the presentation of new ideas, and I thank the scholars who have contributed comments to my conference papers. Those comments have been helpful for me while I wrote the book. I would like to offer my special thanks to Lester Friedman, who, in the context of SCMS, saw the early features of this research and continued to encourage me throughout the book's development.

Colleagues in the Department of Communication at Tulane University gave me my first academic home and shepherded the book through its early stages. I thank Constance Balides, Carole Daruna, Marsha Houston, Ana Lopez, Jim Mackin, Vicki Mayer, John Patton Mauro Porto, Kathleen Turner, Frank Ukadike, and Michele White. Stephen Verderber in the School of Architecture was very generous with his expertise and always made me feel welcome as I explored health care architecture, a terrain that was new to me. Other Tulane staff gave helpful assistance in many ways, and for that I thank Maria Cariana, Marie Davis, Vincent Illustre, Gaye LeMon, Clay McGovern, and David Robinson. My current colleagues in the Department of Media Studies at Queens College, City University of New York, have provided support and friendship through the book's final stages. I give my thanks to Zoe Beloff, Jonathan Buchsbaum, Mara Einstein, Heather Hendershot, Amy Herzog, Anupama Kapse, Stuart Liebman, Susan Macmillan, Richard Maxwell, Leslie McCleave, Roopali Mukherjee, and Ellen Scott. I would also like to take this opportunity to thank my students (too many now to name individually, but their collective presence animates this book's pages) for asking questions and for bringing inquiring and energetic minds to the classroom.

Ken Wissoker, my editor at Duke University Press, saw the potential of my book, kept me on track through the revision process, and gave the perfect balance of encouragement and critical attention that allowed me to transform a manuscript into my first book. He is an excellent editor and a friend. Through his guidance, the anonymous readers engaged with my book in deep, sustained, and meaningful ways. My thanks also go to Courtney Berger and Leigh Barnwell for answering multiple questions and for just being outstanding. Anitra Grisales provided a second pair of fresh editorial eyes when I most needed them.

Some of the ideas presented in chapter 3 appeared in an earlier and different form as "The Nurse-Saver and the TV Hostess: Advertising Hospital Television, 1950–1970," in *Cultural Sutures: Medicine and*

*Media*, ed. Lester Friedman (Durham: Duke University Press, 2004), 73–92. Additionally, a preliminary version of this material also appeared as "You Take Care of the Patients, We'll Take Care of Their TV: Attending to Hospital Television," *Television and New Media* 4, no. 3 (August 2003): 231–56.

I could not have completed this project if it were not for a wonderful network of dedicated friends (some of whom also happen to be really good cooks). For support that has exceeded expectation and for reading multiple versions of chapters and of the entire book, I thank Richard Maxwell, Eileen Meehan, Roopali Mukherjee, Gayle Murchison, Chantal Nadeau, Carol Stabile, Michele White, and the anonymous readers for Duke University Press. Cynthia Chris read and copyedited drafts of the book to the extent that has guaranteed her a special place in my heart as well as in *The Guinness Book of World Records* (or at least it should). Lorrie Strohecker, MD, was incredibly generous in saving and giving me her volumes of the *Journal of the American Medical Association*, the *New England Journal of Medicine, Medical Economics,* and many other physician-directed publications that I otherwise could not have obtained without an arduous endeavor and outright lying. For warm companionship, amazing meals, and remaining an encouraging voice amid revision, Erin Brewer, MD, MPH, has my continuing gratitude. Other friends and colleagues have given me the energy to persevere and just keep writing. They have been bearers of happiness and unfailing senses of humor. Thanks go to Al Babbitt, Rich Cante, Jean Carlomusto, Vanessa Domico, Lisa Duggan, David Gerstner, Mel Giovinco, Stephanie Houston Grey, Loretta Katherine Harmon, Catherine Hodes, John Louis Howard, Heidi Huber, Julia Kuglen, Sam McBride, Kim Perrier, Philip Prock, Gil Rodman, Nic Sammond, Cynthia Schneider, Birgit Schneidmueller, Elizabeth Snyder, Matthew Tinkcom, Elayne Tobin, Mark Unger, Anke Walz, Mark Williams, Barbara White, Patty White, and Ghen Zando-Dennis.

My father, the late Dr. Mack C. Fuqua, and mother, Idaleene Scheu Fuqua, were always very patient with their only daughter. I dedicate my book to them.

Finally, these acknowledgments would be incomplete if I failed to express thanks for my canine companion of ten years, Stella, who passed away just as my book was nearing completion. Always by my side, she taught me that, no matter what deadlines I face, a dog must always be walked.

> *Entertainment offers the image of "something better" to escape into, or something we want deeply that our day-to-day lives don't provide. Alternative hopes, wishes—these are the stuff of utopia, the sense that things could be better, that something other than what is can be imagined and maybe realized.*
> RICHARD DYER, *ENTERTAINMENT AND UTOPIA*

## Introduction

### TELEVISION, HOSPITAL, HOME

The last time my father and I were together was in a hospital room in Tyler, Texas. He was recovering from a complicated surgery, so we passed the time together by watching our favorite television shows on the Food Network. I sat beside his hospital bed as he reclined. We watched perky Rachael Ray prepare her trademark *30 Minute Meals* and my father's favorite, the drawling Paula Deen, make yet another of her down-home delights. When my father was in the hospital, he and I found it difficult to talk directly to each other, so we talked *indirectly* through the television. My father and I shared a love of cooking and baking, and by watching these shows we could feel a sense of that domestic pleasure within a different space. Every now and then, when Rachael or Paula would add an ingredient or do something that my dad did not approve of, he would express his consternation. He would say what he would have done differently and why *his* way would have been better. This was my father, pure and simple: able to focus on one of his passions and withhold other concerns that might have been on his mind. Together, through the television's presence, we talked about cooking; we allowed ourselves, if only for a brief time, to think of *something better* and to distract ourselves with the steps of recipes, measures of ingredients, and pleasures of home cooking. The television programs, set in studio kitchens designed to resemble ordinary home kitchens, temporarily distracted us from our fears and worries. It gave us something to look forward to: returning home to bake our own macaroni and cheese.

Days later, while standing in his kitchen, I was surrounded by his pots and pans, rows of cookbooks and stacks of cooking magazines such as *A Taste of Home* and *Cuisine*, and bottles of prescription medications. Rachael Ray was chatting in the background from the other room, providing a familiar soundtrack for a very different encounter with my father, one based on his *absence* rather than his *presence*. I tell the story of my father's hospitalization not to emphasize the loss that accompanied it, but as a means of commenting on the role that something as apparently trivial as television played in providing even fleeting emotional and perhaps physical relief from a difficult situation.

Television in the hospital has, for more than sixty years, served multiple purposes, just as it has assumed different roles in homes and other spaces. As the television set became a commonplace domestic appliance in American households, it was simultaneously becoming a routine part of the structural environment of modern hospitals. Used in a variety of ways, from patient entertainment to medical education to closed-circuit systems, television's presence in mid-twentieth-century hospitals signaled their technological sophistication. Its own type of palliative care, television enters into medical spaces; in so doing, it transforms our experiences of those spaces and our experiences as patients, visitors, doctors, nurses, and staff. At the same time, watching television in these clinical contexts also reminded patients of home, serving as a medium— a connective channel—between home, family, friends, and the patient's experience of the hospital. In this way, the introduction of television into the mid-twentieth-century hospital contributed to what I will call its *deinstitutionalization*. My particular use of this term refers to aesthetic as well as structural practices of transforming the built environment of hospitals into spaces that are less clinical and more like homes, or even hotels.[1] Hospitals used this image makeover to appeal to a growing population of potential patients, or health care *consumers*.

The patient-television relationship did not and does not end or begin, of course, when the viewer leaves the hospital. As we will see, over time television has been incorporated as a medical device in the home as well. Television, combined with newer digital media technologies such as the personal computer and the Internet, offers medical advice at our fingertips and through multiple screens. Over the years, by making hospitals feel less like institutions and by bringing medical and health-related information into modern homes, television has naturalized its role in the dissemination of medical information, accustomed us to its presence in medical contexts, and acted as an advocate for the consumer-patient. Thus, from its early incorporation into the private hospital room to contemporary direct-to-consumer prescription drug commercials, I argue that television has been critical to three key transformations in the rise of the medical marketplace: the *deinstitutionalization* of the hospital, the *medicalization* of the home, and the development of what I call the *consumer-patient*. *Prescription TV* details these interrelated, sometimes coterminous processes as it traces how television has become a convalescent companion, a trusted and credible source of medical information, and an important implement in the making of the contemporary consumer-patient.

Television is not only a discursive force shaping our individual and cultural ideas about health and illness; it has a material effect on different kinds of public and private spaces. Television, in the context of contemporary hospitals, doctors' offices, or other health care spaces, both conforms to and restructures our experiences of those sites, our perceptions of these spaces, and our ways of regarding television as a health authority. *Prescription TV* shows how television's material presence as an object and its discursive functions (programming, entertainment, information) bridge the gap between home and hospital and promote a vision of consumer-patient autonomy that is, nevertheless, reliant on others (doctors, pharmaceutical corporations, etc.) for health. This book therefore addresses television in its materiality, as an object in a patient's hospital room or in the doctor's office, and its discursivity, in its role as a diagnostic tool in shaping individual and collective consciousness about "health as a meaningful social practice."[2]

One way that health is both an ideology of well-being and a material, meaningful social practice is through the display and incorporation of self-care into daily routines. An obvious example of the ways that health becomes embodied is through media discourses that address us as potential patients, consumers of particular kinds of medicines, recipients of medical treatments, and subjects for the implementation of modes of responsible citizenship.[3] Through television and its many ways of addressing us as potential patients, but framed primarily by a discourse of health care consumerism, we learn to think of ourselves as active agents in caring for ourselves. We learn to regard this care as, first and foremost, *our* responsibility—a responsibility to be performed by self-monitoring, self-regulating neoliberal citizens.

Whether it is in the form of medical dramas, reality makeover programs promising a new, improved version of an existing self, or advertisements that address us as always on the verge of serious illness, television's content—from individual programs to narrowcast cable networks focusing on healthy lifestyles—presents health as a prerequisite for successful and responsible citizenship. The ideal vision promoted through television, which can vary in specific form, nonetheless tends to privilege a subject who is positioned as the active participant of a therapeutic discourse. Moreover, I emphasize that it is not only in television content where one can find an emphasis on therapeutic or health-oriented discourses, but also in the ways that television, as a material object, is situated within specific spaces as a therapeutic or healing device. For example, advertisements for hospital television promoted the therapeutic features of television viewing. Contrary to other discourses that presumed the ill effects of television, these advertisements argued that when viewed in the context of the hospital, television could offer therapeutic distraction and encourage active mental engagement for patients. Once at home, in a different context and with the passing of time, television continues this therapeutic relationship as it addresses viewers as potential patients in need of various treatments and products. In this regard, it would be simplistic to say that television perpetuates therapeutic discourses that are necessarily useless because they are commercial in orientation.

This book engages with incongruities and complexities surrounding the claim that television can be good for what ails you. It engages with the materiality of television, the ways it has been and continues to be used in hospitals and homes as a privileged object with therapeutic value. In the ways I am using the term, *therapeutic value* means that viewers are understood as deriving some benefit from commercials as well as programming, while they are also positioned as specific kinds of consumer-patients. Therapeutic value, then, has economic value in the production of an awareness of ourselves as potential consumers for health care products, including television.

For more than fifty years, researchers, critics in the popular press, and advocacy groups have decried the detrimental effects that television viewing may have on passive, spongelike audiences, particularly children. Social psychologists, sociologists, medical doctors, and mass communication effects scholars have singled out television as a public health menace.[4] Identified as the main culprit responsible for producing all manner of ills, from childhood obesity, aggressive behavior, anxiety, and sleep disorders to adult-onset diabetes and cardiovascular problems, television—even more than video games—seems to be the bad media object.[5] Beginning with television's entrance into the American home, various critics announced concern over the effects of the new medium on gender roles, with special attention focused on children.[6] However, there is a counter-discourse to be found in surprising places: medical and health-related journals and professional publications. From advertisements by television manufacturers, to hospital administrators, to articles written by physicians on the proper films and radio and television programs to show to different kinds of patients, this parallel discourse about television encourages rather than discourages media use, but under deliberately and necessarily circumscribed conditions.[7] Taking a more nuanced and at times contrary approach to social scientific and communication research into the alleged negative effects of television on viewers, this book explores those parallel discourses to analyze how the medium has been positioned therapeutically as one that might actually be good for what ails you. Whether that stance is indeed right or wrong, in one context or another, is not my interest here. Instead, *Prescription TV* focuses on the positioning of media (film, radio, and television) as therapeutic objects in the modern health care system in the United States, and in turn how these products have helped position the consumer-patient.

*Prescription TV* spans approximately one hundred years, from the late 1910s to the early twenty-first century, and accounts for the ways that mass media have been used to educate and entertain viewers, while also constructing lucrative and receptive markets for a burgeoning health-consumer culture. I trace television's entanglement with health care, from hospital film exhibition practices as early as the First World War, to the ways in which particular concepts of health as well as health care products—specifically, prescription pharmaceuticals—are sold to both health care providers and consumer-patients today. As the story unfolds, we see how television itself has also been considered a health care product. In order to map these transitions, I examine what Ellen Seiter calls "a jamboree of television publicity, histories, cable and broadcast schedules, and promotional contests" in order to decipher vast amounts of health and medical commercial messages.[8]

The book's structure is neither linear nor chronological. It does not make a "once television was good, now it's bad" argument. It focuses on ephemeral advertisements and commercials rather than less fleeting and more ubiquitous health-oriented television dramas, news, or reality television and medical programs. Its shape reflects my original scholarly interests that led me to spend many hours in various medical school libraries researching medical, nursing, and pharmaceutical journals about the use of television in medical contexts. As often happens when engaging in archival research, my interest in this project was the result of following different clues. While researching the history of physician-directed pharmaceutical drug advertisements, I noticed articles and editorial commentary about the use of television in medical contexts. Taking my cue from scholars such as Lynn Spigel and Anna McCarthy, who have studied the history of television in domestic and non-domestic contexts, I wondered when and under what circumstances television entered the hospital and other medical spaces. I was fortunate that the university library where I was doing most of my work had complete collections of not only medical journals and magazines, including *Medical Economics*, but also hospital industry trade publications, such as *The Modern Hospital* and *Hospital Management.* Just as useful and fortuitous was the fact that the bound journals included ephemeral advertisements, so that I could trace the history of the ways that television and its antecedent media, such as film and radio, were introduced into hospitals and other medical contexts.

While television advertisements and cable systems are ubiquitous today, I decided to focus my analysis on the decades during which television itself was being introduced into homes and hospitals in the United States, starting in the 1940s. I also realized that before television, film and radio were offered as therapeutic media in hospitals and that this was an important part of the narrative of the "spatial therapeutics" of television, a concept I will theorize in this book.[9] I began to see a connection between my original research project about how physicians were being addressed as unique participants in pharmaceutical marketing, and how early hospital television advertisers directly addressed hospital doctors, staff, and administrators. By extension, the way these advertisers positioned the ideal television viewer-patient resonated with how consumers were also being addressed as idealized consumer-patients, in relation to the prescription drug advertising that appeared decades later. *Prescription TV* teases out these connections across time, questions television's presumed effects on our health, and thus considers the role of television as a therapeutic device in relation to hospitals, homes, and patients.

## APPROACHES TO TELEVISION STUDIES AND HEALTH

Scholarly approaches to television and health, in communication and media studies, have tended to focus on the depictions of physicians, nurses, and hospitals in narrative television programs. Recently, with the proliferation of reality television programs such as the makeover genre, which Brenda R. Weber astutely analyzes, critical attention has been devoted to the roles of patients and or participants in health-related contexts. Moreover, Mimi White, Jane Shattuc, and Joshua Gamson, for example, have considered the role of television talk shows in facilitating therapeutic discourses and encouraging self-regulation through televised confessions.[10] Given that medical and health-related programming and commercials have been staples in television's pantry for decades, and that various genres focusing on these issues proliferate and thrive, it is remarkable that, as Lester Friedman observes, "few scholars focus on the mediations that occur within that process."[11] Television scholars such as Joseph Turow and Robert Thompson explore television's portrayal of doctors in medical dramas, but other aspects of television's relation to health—namely, the roles it serves in medical settings, both as a device for entertainment *and* education—have been left unattended.[12]

Television viewers surely are accustomed to seeing the wonders and worries of contemporary medicine dramatized through narrative broadcast television serials and reality series, such as *General Hospital* (ABC, 1963–present); *Chicago Hope* (CBS, 1994–2000); *ER* (NBC, 1994–2009); *Grey's Anatomy* (ABC, 2005–present); *House, M.D.* (Fox, 2004–present); *St. Elsewhere* (NBC, 1982–88); *The Biggest Loser* (NBC, 2004–present); *Extreme Makeover* (ABC, 2002–7); talk shows such as *Dr. Phil* (CBS, 2002–present); *The Doctors* (CBS, 2008–present); *The Dr. Oz Show* (Fox, 2009–present); or cable networks dedicated to health, such as The Learning Channel or OWN (Oprah Winfrey Network). Earlier medical dramas include *Medic* (NBC, 1954–56); *The Nurses* (CBS, 1962–65); *Dr. Kildare* (NBC, 1961–66); *Marcus Welby, M.D.* (ABC, 1969–76); *Medical Center* (CBS, 1969–76); and *The Bold Ones: The New Doctors* (NBC, 1969–73). Even the declaration "I'm not a doctor, but I play one on TV" has become a clichéd reference to the ways viewers may accept as authoritative those who appear on TV. Our health, the health of others, and the health of the nation are brought to our homes through broadcast and cablecast niche networks, or through Internet websites such as WebMD and pharmaceutical company websites that offer advertisements as information. In addition to television, consumers are addressed as patients through a variety of advertisements and commercial media, such as billboards, magazines, newspapers, bus panels, and prescription drug promotional items (like branded mousepads, pens, and coffee mugs). One of the key modes of address involves the construction of the viewer as a potential patient and the encouragement of cycles of self-diagnosis and self-surveillance.

In relation to the topic of television and health within media studies, textual analyses of individual television texts or programs have predominated. An exemplary study of television's representation of physicians is Turow's examination of the history of such images and the conditions of their production (e.g., how the American Medical Association influenced television depictions of physicians). To date, however, there are few book-length examinations of either institutional uses of television in health care contexts or television's role in the structuring of health consumerism. This absence may be due, in part, to the dominance of television studies that foreground the home, as well as certain received ways of theorizing consumerism as primarily a leisure-based activity done by nonprofessional female consumers at first-order retail shopping malls. Karen Riggs's ethnography of television in the lives of elderly viewers and McCarthy's analysis of the function of television in, among other places, physicians' waiting rooms, as well as feminist analyses of medical technologies, are examples of this approach to television and its relation to viewers and places.[13] Scholars such as Sander Gilman, Alan M. Kraut, and Judith Walzer Leavitt have engaged in rich historical and cultural analyses of the relationship between medicine and power.[14] Additionally, there have been studies of how television has represented HIV/AIDS and other illnesses, from scholars who are working in the interdisciplinary tradition of cultural studies. Not specifically engaging with the topic of television and health, various scholars have addressed the dynamic between these two elements and have analyzed the ways that particular televisual images and narratives have reinforced or contested dominant meanings about HIV/AIDS.[15] It is my goal to contribute to a conversation *across* fields—from television studies, to the medical humanities, to cultural studies—in order to connect scholarly work that seems contained within its own disciplinary domain.

Within the field of health communication, analyses of media and health examine how health experts present messages to the public (e.g., about antismoking treatments). These studies tend to rely on quantitative measures of the success of health messages or campaigns, with less attention paid to how particular ideas about health may actually prevent or discourage certain individuals and communities from seeking available health care. These approaches, primarily based in quantitative and content analyses, are structured by social scientific considerations of the effects of television on specific kinds of behavior.[16] Offered either as correctives to bad behaviors or criticism of inaccurate mass media images (and positive versus negative imagery), these studies do not account for the ways that specific mass media and their viewers make sense of these messages.

In contrast to the health communication approach to television and health that tends toward a quantitative orientation, other television and media scholars analyze television in ways that challenge both a media-effects mode of understanding and content-based approaches to television programming. While television studies has undergone what some scholars have called a spatial turn and now also considers what television means in places outside the home, it has most often situated television as a domestic medium. Yet, as McCarthy shows in *Ambient Television*, since its earliest moments, television has had a rich life *outside* the home. Moreover, McCarthy argues that the "position of the TV set" in places outside the home, such as retail establishments, taverns, or even physicians' waiting rooms, also "helps to position people ... within the social organization of the space[s] and within larger networks of power, as well."[17] This kind of double positioning is especially relevant for mapping television's uses—and the ways viewers are asked to regard it—within health care environments and in domestic spaces.

*Prescription TV* analyzes the role that television and other media have played in the repositioning not only of the domestic space of the home as a primary site of medical care, but also of the consuming subject as, first and foremost, a potential patient. My book traces the role of media in the construction of the modern medical marketplace, and its implications, in the United States. *Prescription TV* responds to a neglected area in the theorization of consumer culture and television through an examination of health consumerism and medical media, and engages with both media studies and the growing interdisciplinary field of the medical humanities.[18] For example, while studies of consumer culture have tended to privilege shopping as the primary consumption form, my book challenges this assumption by examining other practices, such as health consumerism, that may not be readily described through the existing theoretical frameworks. A more productive way to think about the ways health is marketed to us through a convergence of education and entertainment is to acknowledge that, like all forms of consumption, there is a desired outcome or reason for us to purchase the product. Moreover, health care consumerism is similar to other forms of consumerism that are more recognizably leisure based. While it may be the case that some consumers shop as if their lives depended on it, with health-related goods and services, outright dismissals of consumerism for its sheer impulsiveness become more complicated to make. It is, moreover, important to ask how health-related products (like prescription drugs) are similar to or different from other commercial commodities, but it is just as important to ask how and for whom these products matter.

Television, professional and popular magazines, websites and blogs, celebrity testimonials, and technologies of home safety and patient monitoring work together to privilege a new kind of patient: a consumer that, under the rules of neoliberal ideology applied to health, is responsible for his or her own health or illness. This may take the shape of a "care of the self" in which one's body is literally remade according to normative ideals of beauty or health.[19] The reconstruction of the body to locate the true self, as Weber indicates, is neither simply passive nor representative of independent "self-making."[20] Rather, to take the example of the ways that bodies are remade through the ubiquitous makeover reality television genre, this mode of subjectivity participates within a "makeover nation" that is structured by neoliberal tenets supporting "a version of the good and proper citizen as one who is self-aware, an active participant in consumer culture," and who "performs such maintenance of the self ostensibly as a free agent with the state exempted from social welfare responsibilities."[21]

### USES OF TELEVISION IN THE HOSPITAL AND OTHER MEDICAL CONTEXTS

*Prescription TV* is less focused on television content than on its various uses and functions within medical and health-related contexts. While it is the case that there is much about television to be critical of—from its stereotypical depictions of race, class, and gender to its economic structure—my aim is to offer a history of the medium that has yet to be told: the role it has played, and continues to play, in clinical spaces, along with its function as a key component of the ever-expanding medicalization of everyday life. In the following pages, I resituate television in terms of its status as the scrutinized object—particularly in relation to health care institutions and industries—and as a participant in the construction of the contemporary medical marketplace. Toward that end, I engage questions of television and health from the other side of the debate about the medium's assumed effects. Television's capacity to do something other than harm its viewers is one of the book's central themes. In fact, on its own television does little; however, we as consumer-patients of a variety of mediated health messages do many things with television and use its texts in ways that are meaningful and unpredictable.

The Healium Network is one example of how television is used in a medical context to keep patients' minds off the time spent waiting to see physicians, while it also facilitates a cozy relationship between medical information and medical marketing. The subscription cable network provides original programming that focuses on what it calls patient education, about such topics as tort reform, the latest pharmaceutical breakthroughs, and healthy lifestyle features. It also runs "feel good" segments from shows such as *Entertainment Tonight* and *Dr. Phil*, news segments from *60 Minutes*, and classic situation comedies such as *I Love Lucy* and *The Honeymooners*. The Healium Network's parent entity is AVTV Networks, which provides "stress-free" programming and "entertainment over education because that's what patients in waiting rooms prefer." The goal of the Healium Network is to "relax and entertain patients while they are in the waiting room."[22]

If the Healium Network's intent is to help patients pass the time in doctors' offices, then when patients are in hospitals, television is assumed to have a similar function. One of the structuring assumptions about television's presence in patient rooms or hospital or medical office waiting areas is that, in these contexts, television viewing can be a positive thing. Why? It has the potential to distract us from pain, boredom, or other stress- and anxiety-producing states. On the other hand, it also has, as Robert Crawford argues, the potential to induce stress and anxiety.[23] Moreover, television content in explicitly medical contexts tends to be space appropriate and narrowcast, so that the programming is specifically produced for patients. This, however, is not a new development; hospitals have been producing original programming since the early 1950s through closed-circuit television systems, with nurses, physicians, and staff serving as producers, directors, and performers. Some of the earliest examples of hospital television programming included closed-circuit instruction for new mothers in how to bathe and care for their infants. Television in hospitals has always been more than an entertainment device. In addition to providing patients with the same programs that their families and friends might be watching at home, hospital television was used to educate patients about how to care for themselves and others.

While television can and should be critiqued for many reasons, rarely do television's detractors delve deeper into the economic structure of television to account for its content, structure, and organization. Nor do they ask why other sedentary forms of leisure, such as reading, writing, knitting, or playing board games, are not critiqued with the same force. The formulation of the passive television viewer tends to equate physical stillness with mental inactivity. In some cases, particularly if the viewer is required to be physically inactive due to illness, stillness might be preferred. If it is the case, as my book argues, that physical inactivity does not equal mental passivity, then what other questions does this allow us to ask about our relationship to television?

### KEYWORDS: DEINSTITUTIONALIZATION, MEDICALIZATION, AND THE CONSUMER-PATIENT

Raymond Williams, in his introduction to *Keywords*, reminds us that it is not enough to study the origin of a word, or the context of its use over time—its use in life—but that it is also incumbent on the theorist or historian to recognize "as any study of language must, that there is indeed community between past and present, but also that community—that difficult word—is not the only possible description of these relations between past and present; that there are also radical change, discontinuity and conflict, and that all these are still at issue and are indeed still occurring."[24] It is in this spirit of communities of meanings that I offer these remarks about three of the main keywords of this book. They are touchstones through which ideologies and material practices converge and extend; they allow different ways of imagining both what it could mean to be a patient, and the role that television plays in this process.

To assert that television has played a central role in the "deinstitutionalization" of modern hospitals while, at the same time, that it helped transform homes into privatized medical clearinghouses offering a plethora of health-related information, raises the following questions: How has this dual transformation been accomplished? And what are the consequences? When I use the term *deinstitutionalization*, I do not intend to suggest that hospitals and other health care facilities such as doctor's offices are no longer institutions in the sense of being complex economic and bureaucratic structures that function hierarchically and are governed by many different types of local, state, and federal policies and legal regulations. While remaining institutions in this broad sense, however, at least since the second decade of the twentieth century, hospital administrators and physicians in the United States increasingly have been concerned not only with the sanitary or hygienic conditions of their medical facilities, but also with the aesthetic features and experiential attributes of hospitals and clinics. The deinstitutionalization I am interested in has more to do with the perception of institutionalized spaces of care rather than with an actual, structural change in the functioning of hospitals, insurance companies, federal medical welfare programs, and physicians. While it is indeed the case that the institutionalized medical system in the United States warrants a significant revision, I am focusing on how hospital and health care administrators, as representatives of institutions, attempted to shift public perception of hospitals from that of cold, clinical spaces to centers of personalized and comfortable care. This was accomplished, this book argues, less through actual changes in hierarchical structure and protocol than through the adoption of architectural and design changes along with the incorporation of patient-centered media and marketing.

Just as television helped to deinstitutionalize hospitals, it contributed to the medicalization of the modern home and the maintenance of the self. "Medicalization" is a concept that designates a process through which "medicine, with its distinctive ways of thinking, models, metaphors, and institutions comes to exercise authority over areas of life not previously considered medical."[25] As physicians at the close of the nineteenth and beginning of the twentieth centuries were staking out their professional ground and authority over health and illness, attendant institutions, structures, practices, and ideas were also building on the ideas promulgated by modern medicine. One of the hallmarks of medicalization is that it encourages people to think differently about themselves, to regard their bodies in different ways, and to think of themselves as, first and foremost, potential patients.

A second key feature of medicalization recasts personal or social problems in terms of health and illness, and poses medical solutions to problems that might otherwise be addressed through a change in our social and professional roles as mothers, fathers, daughters, sons, wives, husbands, spouses, partners, citizens, and workers. Further, medicalizing certain problems, feelings, or ways of understanding or conceptualizing the social world may prevent us from approaching the situation from any other perspective. Medicalization is about control and interpretation. For example, rather than imagining how particular situations may be changed or symptoms lessened through nonmedical means, a battery of prescription medicines are consumed. What can be overlooked by such a description of medicalization is that it tends to disregard the limitations on individual agency that may make it extremely difficult for a patient to change, either interpersonally or socially. It may not be possible for the individual to address a situation without assistance—from chemical or other more conventional talk-therapeutic sources. Moreover, if a patient should need help from prescription drugs to address daily problems, does this make him or her less worthy or significant than someone who can manage his or her problems on their own? In a culture where pulling oneself up by one's bootstraps seems to function as a commonsense mandate, this makes seeking any kind of help—much less help in the form of prescription drugs—seem like an indication of personal weakness or failure.

The phenomenon described by the term *medicalization* is historical. As scholars such as Adele Clarke, Paula Treichler, Lisa Cartwright, Leonore Tiefer, and Catherine Waldby suggest, medicalization may more appropriately denote an era of professionalization.[26] This era has included the continued professionalization of medicine and the legitimation of various support professions. The next phase of growth in this phenomenon includes a deeper penetration of medical authority and understanding into people's everyday lives, referred to as *biomedicalization*.[27]

Regarding the convergence and divergence of medicalization and biomedicalization, Clarke and colleagues further suggest that both moments may exist at the same time and that they are mutually defining. Each continues to function both distinctly and always in relation to the other.[28] That is, from the dazzle of diagnostic imaging machines to the neoliberal, market-driven consumerist mode of health care in which health itself becomes a commodity, these two modes of medicine and science/technology can be seen in today's medical marketplace. As these processes are occurring, the meaning and role of the state in relation to the governed is under radical revision, as the relentless policies and economies of neoliberalism work in tandem with biomedicalization to generate consumer-patients—the ideal of the self-regulating, self-monitoring citizen. This citizen is one who is compliant while seeming autonomous, controlled through the discourse of choice, and governed through self-reliance and self-surveillance. Television, this book argues, plays a central role in the discursive production of health identities through which consumer-patients are encouraged to live their lives.

The third term that structures this book is a merger of what were once two distinct categories: the patient and the consumer. At least since the 1980s, when the market-based language of consumer choice began to be used by health insurance companies, health care facilities, and other health industry constituencies, the idea of what it means to be a patient has been radically redefined from that of passive recipient of medical care to that of the active, information-seeking consumer-patient. Assuming that the medical industry functions like other markets and that patients have the choice to select primary care physicians (from a circumscribed list provided by their insurance carriers—if they have insurance), the language of the marketplace has supplanted, for all intents and purposes, the more altruistic, less economically driven language of earlier doctor-patient relationships. While, to a degree, the replacement of the patient by the consumer represents a reaction against paternalistic, ideological constructs of the patient as the passive recipient of expert care, it also now suggests that patients are indeed endowed with the same kinds of (limited) choice as other kinds of consumers and are free to determine their own health care treatments—and, by extension, their own health outcomes.[29] This is far from the case, as the following chapters will show.

The medical historian Nancy Tomes argues that the first users of the term *health-care consumer* were not "market enthusiasts," but "patient activists" in the 1960s and '70s who were "part of a wide-ranging critique of both medical paternalism and the 'new medical industrial complex.'" Tomes uses the term *patient/consumer* to indicate the historical, economic, and political shift from one model of the complex relationship between patients, physicians, and the medical industrial complex, to another model based more on market ideas of individual choice and competitive quality. What initially started out as a positive political and discursive intervention in the ways that patients understood their position in relation to power structures (embodied by physicians and other medical authorities and experts) has now been corrupted by consumer-driven market modes. While some medical historians of health care policy see the replacement of the patient model by the consumer model as at least a potentially positive indication of an increase in patient power and self-determination, Tomes argues that this shift in nomenclature and also the rise of consumer-based advocacy groups "are best understood as responses to long-term *contractions*, not *expansions* of patients' powers of therapeutic and economic" autonomy. Tomes's use of the patient/consumer reflects a historical shift from passive patient to active consumer, yet she argues that while there have been significant changes in the ways that patients and physicians understand their roles in terms of expertise and self-determination, the balance of power, based on the structure of the marketplace, actually works more to the advantage of medical entrepreneurs by making "medicine more business-like."[30] That is, by marketing prescription drugs to patients, by making health care facilities seem less like institutions (or businesses) and more like friendly spaces of individualized treatment, or by enabling patients to achieve increased levels of expertise and knowledge about their own bodies and health, it might be possible to actually produce empowered patients rather than patient/consumers, as Tomes suggests.

Some health care scholars have also argued that the logic of market-based approaches to health care cannot be successful because as patients we do not select our physician or our treatments for conditions and illnesses like we select other goods and services—"on the basis of price and quality."[31] Yet, increasingly, we as consumer-patients *do* (for those who have the privilege of health care) engage with health care choices based on price, perceived quality, and many other factors. These choices may indeed be limited and may be made on the basis of marketing rather than information, or a combination of the two. But we always engage with these choices as both consumers *and* patients. It certainly is the case that the medical marketplace sees our lives in terms of profit and price, often over considerations of quality and care. Consumer-patients embody a complex position. They represent a history of the change from passive patient to a patient with at least a certain kind of agency—even if this agency is largely inscribed and delimited by the medical marketplace.[32]

Rather than adopt Tomes's term of *patient/consumer*, which indicates a historical progression from passive patient to active consumer, I have used the term *consumer-patient* to call attention to their conflation. As Tomes indicates, it is best not to "jettison the language of the empowered patient/consumer until we have a better alternative in place."[33] Indeed, consumer-patient, as I use it throughout the book, directs attention to the limitations as well as the possibilities of such a co-constituent subject. Whereas Tomes's use of the term *patient/consumer* implies a possible distinction, consumer-patient works against that possibility and recognizes that we are both consumers *and* patients in this medical marketplace.

The five chapters and conclusion that follow represent a range of approaches to the key concepts elaborated in this introduction. From a historical examination of how entertainment media such as film, radio, and television have been used as healing devices in different kinds of health care contexts, to an analysis of the rise of one of the most obvious examples of consumer-patient medical marketing—prescription drug television commercials—the book examines how television has figured in each of the key transformations represented by the *deinstitutionalization* of hospitals, the *medicalization* of the modern home, and the construction of the *consumer-patient*.[34] Elaborating a series of material and discursive processes and texts through which viewer health is increasingly understood and mediated via televisual systems, the book concludes with an exploration of what is at stake in the dissolution of the divide between professional expertise and patients, hospitals and home. By focusing on the ways that television has functioned both outside the home in medical contexts, and inside the home as a medical information center, *Prescription TV* foregrounds the continuities between these spaces.[35]

In order to comprehend the conditions under which television entered hospitals in the United States during the late 1940s, it is necessary to understand the history of the ways that earlier media were administered to patients. Chapter 1 examines earlier forms of patient entertainment, including film and radio, and the guiding assumptions that shaped therapeutic care and the processes of medicalization. Interestingly, while advocates of film regulation and censorship were protesting the apparently harmful effects of cinema spectatorship, companies such as Eastman Kodak were busy encouraging hospital administrators to transform their wards and private patient rooms into film exhibition sites. This chapter, as well as the ones that follow, relies on historical advertisements and trade industry articles that document how entertainment media were understood to have therapeutic properties—administered under controlled circumstances, of course. These advertisements and other textual evidence from the health industry press allow us to see how television was eventually adopted in these spaces, and to understand how hospital personnel and film equipment manufacturers regarded the relationship between patients and spectatorship. In many ways, film spectatorship and radio listening in hospitals complicate accepted ideas about both the contexts of exhibition and the condition of spectators. This chapter maps the ways that these two different media, film and radio, paved the way for television as a therapeutic device. While there are instances of physicians making films of their patients and of certain surgical procedures, during the late 1910s and 1920s film was most often used for patient entertainment.[36] Likewise, radio was sometimes combined with nurse-call communication systems, at least in its early installation in hospitals, though it was first used as a hospital amenity for patients. As precedents for television, film and radio were brought into the spaces of hospitals in the United States as ways of deinstitutionalizing potentially foreboding structures, and to comfort patients.

Continuing the history of hospital deinstitutionalization and the media, chapter 2 chronicles the incorporation of television into the architecture, functioning, and advertising of the mid-twentieth-century hospital. This chapter focuses on the architectural history of television's placement in hospitals to look at the ways that television both reconfigured and challenged the material structures of hospitals. As hospitals attempted to sell the public on the idea of the modern institution, full of the latest technological and scientific diagnostic devices, hospital administrators used television to inject familiarity into an otherwise unfamiliar context. In the modern hospital, television offered the promise of connecting patients to the outside world; it also created a sense of continuity between patients' homes and their hospital experiences. But television was used not only for patient entertainment and "video visits," but also as closed-circuit systems for the transmission of live surgical procedures for medical student audiences, and for nurse-produced, in-house hospital programs for new mothers. This architectural and spatial analysis of television's installation in hospitals reveals the medium's central position in the development and transformation of institutional practices of health care and the rise of modern health consumerism.

Television's utility in the hospital, both as a medical device itself and as an attractive accessory, was not a given. Chapter 3 thus extends the history of television installation in hospitals through an examination of the ways that television manufacturers sold hospital administrators and patients on the idea of therapeutic TV. I argue that using what I call *spatial therapeutics*, advertisements for hospital television marketed their product, first and foremost, as a therapeutic medium and as a necessary piece of hospital equipment. These advertisements can be seen as blueprints that depict preferred configurations for television within the individual patient's room, and also for the placement of the patient in relation to the television. The patient's bed and the television become focal points in the advertisements, which often do not feature any other medical equipment. Through an analysis of the ways that television is positioned within the context of the patient room and the ways that patients are positioned in relation to the television, we see how advertisers manipulated spatial therapeutics and notions of patient agency to sell their product. Chapter 3 examines the representation of television as a spatially therapeutic medium within the patient room, and shows how patients are positioned as viewers who are both compliant and endowed with agency over at least a part of their hospital experience.

The first three chapters of *Prescription TV* show how film, radio, and television manufacturers sold hospital administrators on the idea of entertainment media as one way to deinstitutionalize modern hospitals. As part of that process, strong connections between the hospital and the home, as well as the patient and the consumer, began to emerge. The next two chapters extend those links by focusing on how pharmaceutical marketing and other aspects of contemporary medical consumerism have helped medicalize the modern home and further interpolate the consumer-patient. Chapters 4 and 5 examine the development of health consumerism, the medicalization of the modern home, and the rise of television advertising to both doctors and consumer-patients, by investigating the economic and ideological aspects of commercial health discourse on television. Taking a case-study approach to the phenomenon of medicalization and the rise of the consumer-patient, these two chapters tell two interrelated stories about media and health consumerism.

Chapter 4 sets the historical backdrop for the 1997 television debut of prescription drug commercials aimed at consumers. For nearly one hundred years before the appearance of direct-to-consumer drug commercials, physicians were the primary target market for pharmaceutical manufacturers. As the initial audience of pharmaceutical industry address, physicians have constituted one of the most powerful markets for the promotion and circulation of prescription drugs. Marketing practices such as physician detailing as well as physician-aimed advertisements in medical journals, pharmaceutical industry–funded medical research protocols, and other means of influencing physicians' prescribing behavior, paved the way for the development of direct-to-consumer drug advertising and the positioning of the consumer-patient. This chapter lays the historical and regulatory groundwork to account for prescription drug advertising on television and anticipates the case study in chapter 5 of one ubiquitous prescription drug, Pfizer's Viagra.

During any portion of daytime and primetime television, we can find commercials for a range of prescription drugs. Charles Acland has argued that "drugs are a site of *micropower*; they condense and reproduce exacting relations of power among the fields of industry, medicine, and bodies."[37] Prescription drug ads specifically marketed to men generally place them in outdoor and group contexts, engaging in typically masculine activities. In chapter 5, I analyze the Viva Viagra and NASCAR campaigns to demonstrate the ways that Pfizer uses intertextual humor to market what's known as the "little blue pill." This final chapter condenses the key concepts that animate this book—deinstitutionalization, medicalization, and the consumer-patient—while it also extends its reach to engage with a specific form of consumer-patient subject positioning: that of the aging male.

While I do not analyze television programming content in this book, I do attend to discourses about and images of television in medical contexts and as a medical product. Thus, in this final chapter, I turn my attention to television commercials. Prescription drug commercials are watched in a variety of contexts, just as advertisements for Viagra and other brand-name drugs are seen in subway cars, billboards, magazines, and bus stops. Yet I focus my examination of these commercial forms and companion Internet websites as if they are targeting a likely viewer consuming these segments in the comfort of his or her home. As home becomes a site for the implementation of medical care and an accessible medical research archive via websites such as WebMD, it becomes increasingly difficult to argue that we, as consumer-patients, are unsophisticated dupes of the medical marketplace. It is more to the point to say that while consumer-patients are amalgamated subjectivities and no doubt positioned in relation to specific regulating discourses, we are also becoming ever more attuned to the implications of healthy subjectivity—for ourselves and for others. In some cases, healthy subjectivity suggests an internalization of neoliberal self-regulation and control, yet it never means just one thing. Indeed, combinations of commerce and culture, education and information, mediate our ideas about the healthy self.

*Prescription TV* concludes with an analysis of how consumer-patients are actually becoming the material of television. Not simply in front of the screen, consumer-patients now occupy the position of personalized witness to the technoscientific wonders of modern medicine. One way this is happening is through reality programming that focuses on health, bodies, and self-improvement. Far from being a mere distraction or serving only educational purposes, health has become the substance of entertainment itself.

## Convalescent Companions
### HOSPITAL ENTERTAINMENT BEFORE TELEVISION

Motion pictures and radio preceded television's entrance into hospitals in the United States by more than thirty years. In order to more fully account for television in the hospital, as a *new* technology in an *established* space, it is important to understand the technological and cultural frameworks that facilitated the incorporation of the new media technology. Indeed, as these forms of new media entered into the established, institutional spaces of hospitals, they helped create what we recognize as the modern hospital. While curing and treating disease, performing surgeries, and delivering babies were and continue to be the main features of a hospital's function, another aspect of patient care involves providing a healing environment that offers therapeutic leisure for the mind and the body. As film, radio, and later television found their places in various viewing and listening contexts, hospitals adapted these entertainment media to the specificities of patient need, comfort, and hygiene. Hospitals also employed media to establish a new way of thinking about the hospital as a clinical space, as well as what it means to be a patient within that space.[1]

As a form of therapeutic distraction, film exhibition in hospitals had its debut during the last two years of the First World War. In military hospitals in the United States and France, wounded soldiers were shown American films for entertainment. Later, as American hospitals began to modernize and revise the institutional, cold, and unpleasant clinical characteristics of hospitals, film and radio were used to signify both modern technology and a homelike environment. By 1920 some hospitals in the United States were showing movies, and in 1923 radio was introduced at Beth Israel Hospital in New York City. Films were shown in both private rooms and wards, just as radio sets were placed so that many patients could listen either in a group setting or, after the introduction of headsets, alone. Film and radio quickly became used as therapeutic and educational devices that simultaneously distracted patients from the experience of being in the hospital, while also reminding them of life elsewhere, beyond the hospital.

This chapter tells the story of how film, and just a few years later, radio, came to be recognized as *therapeutic* media, helping to provide spectators and listeners with corporeal experiences that were defined, at least potentially, more by *pleasure* than by *pain*. As a demonstration of media geography and as a historicization of the place(s) of media technology, this chapter explains how film and radio were introduced into the institutional realm of hospitals in the United States, establishing a framework for television's entrance during the early 1950s. Among other forces that helped institutionalize the therapeutic uses of media in medical settings, such as programs that facilitated the projection of films in military and civilian hospitals, early advertisements for film and radio devices played a key role in establishing the idea that media could be used as therapeutic tools in the hospital. Articulating a discourse that sometimes seemed at odds with popular press and research studies about the presumed harmful effects of film and radio, during the 1920s film production and distribution companies such as the Eastman Kodak Company Medical Division, along with radio and sound reproduction manufacturers like Western Electric, represented their media products as just what the doctor ordered.[2]

Early advertisements for film and radio in hospitals touted the perceived therapeutic benefits of media consumption by repositioning the patient as a mentally active, yet perhaps physically immobile, film spectator or radio listener. These advertisements from the 1920s underscore that, at least from the perspective of film and radio manufacturers and hospital personnel, media consumption is not passive. This is emphasized through the ways the patient is positioned in the advertisements, and how the instructions for media use assume the patient is mentally active and engaged while being, to varying degrees, physically inactive or at least limited in his or her physical movements. Thus these advertisements support contemporary media theorists' and critics' arguments that media consumption is not now and never has been passive. Even while inactive because of illness or accident, patients can, to greater or lesser degrees, respond and engage with media.

By the early 1920s, with motion pictures drawing large crowds to movie palaces, hospitals began to ponder the possibilities of bringing home movies and other entertainment films to inpatients. As we will see with the case of hospital television, the implicit assumption that structured the promotion of film spectatorship and radio listening in the hospital was that, at least within the confines of that space, film and media could be their own form of therapeutic entertainment. Patients, through in-hospital media consumption, could feel connected to the outside world and their ordinary lives. Film projection programs and advertisements for hospital film and radio not only promised to keep patients in a therapeutic frame of mind, but to create a different experience of the hospital as a clinical space, and a different way to be a patient within that space. Articles in trade publications like *The Modern Hospital*, directed to hospital administrators, specifically addressed the issue of how to make hospitals more hospitable for their middle-class patients.[3] These types of historical documents demonstrate how the introduction of motion pictures into hospitals went hand in hand with the transformation of modern hospitals from places of last resort to places that represented the powers of scientific medicine.[4] Watching films and listening to radio in hospitals naturalized their role in these contexts, while the presence of media entertainment facilitated the deinstitutionalization of clinical space.

Among the historical materials I analyze here are advertisements for film and radio. They are rich historical texts, not only for the information they provide about the ideal consumers of the featured commodities, but also for how they represent certain cultural and economic assumptions about media. As prescriptions for ideal uses and functions within particular spaces, advertisements can offer clues as to the ways that manufacturers of portable film projectors and radios assumed that their products could be incorporated into hospital and home settings.[5] Indeed, advertisements appearing in professional and trade publications related to medical care and health tell us as much about the place of film, radio, and television within hospitals and clinical sites as they do about the ideal spectators, listeners, and viewers. Moreover, the specificity of the marketing discourse directed toward hospitals constructs a vision of healthy mass media that is at odds with critical debates about their role in society. These particular examples also underscore how film, radio, and television advertisers were responding to a new market—hospitals. Therefore, this chapter focuses on advertisements and attendant articles as key discursive frames for the analysis of media's assumed role within hospitals, about the hopes and hesitations that accompanied their use in these spaces, and the relief they may have provided.

The documents used in this chapter include advertisements and articles from a range of trade, professional, and consumer publications spanning the years 1918 to 1932. I examine advertisements and articles from *The Moving Picture World* and *Radio Retailing*, two trade publications; *The Modern Hospital*, a publication addressed to medical professionals like hospital administrators; and *Hygeia*, the consumer magazine published by the American Medical Association. These publications make clear the ways that, from administrative, industrial, and consumer perspectives, pre-television media such as film and radio were incorporated into hospital routines and spaces, and the attendant assumptions that guided their reception. *The Modern Hospital*, *The Moving Picture World*, and *Radio Retailing* represent concerns with media and health care from an inside perspective that allows us to understand how and under which administrative, economic, and spatial circumstances such media entered hospitals.

## MOVIES AS MEDICINE

As the First World War unfolded, ideas regarding the function and purpose of American hospitals began changing. In short, hospitals needed to create a certain perception of indispensability and accessibility on the part of non-medical personnel. A variety of factors worked together to transform hospitals in the United States. Some of these factors included "hospital budgets, physician's practice patterns, attitudes toward science, charity, and the prerogatives of class—as well as the X-ray, antiseptic surgery, and clinical laboratories."[6] Moreover, "From the 1870s on, hospitals had sought to present an inviting and increasingly *scientific* image to the public. In annual reports and planted newspaper stories, they underlined two themes: first, that their private rooms offered the comfort and convenience of a hotel with the ambience of a home; and second, that professional care and a newly effective technology could only be provided in a hospital."[7] In addition to gleaming medical equipment, the *display* of modern communication technologies and interior design signified a hospital's legitimacy, capability, and care.[8] Through the production of a *homelike atmosphere*, modern hospitals represented themselves as *familiar* places devoted to the "care of strangers."[9] Other hospitals tried to produce, through interior design, the atmosphere of modern hotels.[10] Hospitals engaged in a variety of practices to show that they could provide levels of care and comfort that were better than those in all but the wealthiest of private homes. One of these practices involved introducing film projection in the hospital.

An early example of films shown for patient entertainment occurred during the First World War. Films were shown on transport and battleships, as well as at the front lines of conflict in Red Cross and YMCA recreation huts and hospitals. Under the guidance of Mrs. Dunham Foster, of the New York City–based Community Motion Picture Bureau, and her staff, extra care was taken to match film genres to particular aspects of military operations.[11] Films that would not "work too much on their feelings" were shown to soldiers at embarkation points, while lighthearted comedies or romances were shown at battlefronts and in hospitals.[12] Movies as medicine, however, were not limited to battlefront contexts, but were also beneficial to soldiers in hospitals. Movies shown to recovering soldiers varied from entertainment to educational films, but the context determined which kinds of films were shown to which patients.

Concern for soldiers' morale and morals regarding entertainment extended to the highest levels of military command, with General J. J. Pershing ordering the U.S. Army to provide the troops with uplifting entertainment. As General Pershing, in 1918, said to E. C. Carter, the general secretary of the YMCA in Paris (its European headquarters for the entertainment operation), "Morale is a state of mind upheld by entertainment."[13] Entertainment, in this case, was used as a kind of moralistic prophylactic to discourage soldiers from pursuing foreign pleasures and to encourage their fighting spirits. When soldiers were injured, U.S. Army–approved entertainment was used to heal broken bodies and soothe shell-shocked minds.

Supporting the perceived importance of therapeutic film viewing, new projection techniques were developed in order to adapt to patients needs. As *The Modern Hospital* noted, patients limited to lying on their backs could not see projected films. So "portable motion-picture machines are stationed so that the projections appear on the ceiling, and all the patient lying on his back need do is to look up."[14] The hospital context, at once private and public, both a site for the care of the ill as well as a place of work and visitation for the well, required certain technological (formal) and cultural (content) adaptations. The earliest documentation of the exhibition of film in hospitals for the designated purpose of patient entertainment comes from September 1918. Indeed, many of the ideas about the restorative, therapeutic qualities of film, and later radio and television, in hospitals and other institutional health care facilities can be traced to the use of motion pictures for military entertainment and for wounded soldiers. During and at the close of the First World War, never had the medical infrastructure of the United States been asked to care for so many sick and wounded individuals.

From the perspective of medical professionals and hospital personnel, movies played a key role in therapeutic practices not only in military hospitals, but in civilian ones as well. Some of the structuring assumptions that brought movies to hospitals were that film spectatorship could be enjoyed by many different kinds of patients and that, if need be, specific films could be shown to specific patients. Film, silent during the early years of hospital projection, was also, compared to other entertainment activities such as reading, an experience that could accommodate a group or be shown to an individual patient. If patients were dealing with diminished or restricted physical capacities, then the movies could provide entertaining mental distraction with minimal physical effort. What is interesting from a medical perspective is how doctors, nurses, and hospital staff recognized that the movies were highly adaptable to the hospital routine, and that there was something specific to the medium with therapeutic potential. For one thing, film spectatorship in the hospital, like theatrical film spectatorship, facilitated discussion among the spectators. It allowed people who may not have anything else to say to one another the opportunity to share an experience and to talk about it afterward. It also allowed the spectators to laugh together and discuss topics other than their immediate personal discomfort or pain. In order for films to enter the hospital context, medical personnel had to recognize this capacity of film to facilitate conversation and to give patients a respite from their personal discomfort through the narrative pleasures of the movies.

## "HOSPITAL HAPPINESS"

As a test of the hospital as a site for film exhibition and patient pleasure, George Eastman started the "Hospital Happiness Movement" in 1920 in Rochester, New York. This movement facilitated film exhibition for patients at all the hospitals in Rochester on a weekly schedule.[15] This therapeutic and marketing experiment proved successful, and in just a few years, the Eastman Kodak Company Medical Division began targeting hospital administrators across the United States as potential markets for its films, projectors, and screens.[16] The Hospital Happiness Movement was "supported by the contributions of moving picture patrons, deposited in the boxes in the lobbies of motion picture houses throughout Rochester."[17] In this way, conventional theatrical exhibition actually supported and facilitated non-theatrical film spectatorship. *The Modern Hospital* endorsed the Hospital Happiness Movement and understood film spectatorship to be a suitable form of entertainment that could "be enjoyed without exertion by all who are in a condition to enjoy anything."[18] Film spectatorship, from a clinical perspective, was therapeutic because it did not require physical exertion, though it did require that a patient be able to see.

Even if the patient was blind, however, it could be possible for other patients to narrate the story. The idea that film spectatorship was therapeutic, partly because it did not require physical movement, structured the use of film in hospitals. Perhaps because film spectatorship does not require the viewer to turn pages in a book, lift one's head, or otherwise move the body, this form of entertainment was understood as especially adaptable for patients. In this case, the film industry, as represented by Eastman, stresses the inactive physical state of the patient—but only temporarily so—as a form of spectator therapy. If the patient is incapable of moving, or at least is diminished physically, then film as a form of therapy facilitates the return of normative health through mental activity.

The Hospital Happiness Movement is significant for several reasons, both in terms of how entertainment was perceived clinically and for what it shows us about early issues of projection and reception. First, it shows how hospital administrators regarded film not only in terms of its material aspects (how to project images, which types of materials could be used as makeshift screens, etc.) but also with regard to its social functions. That is, if theatrical film spectatorship was a social event, then this was also the case in terms of hospital film exhibition and spectatorship.

Implicit in the incorporation of motion pictures into this institutional context was the idea that the hospital was more than simply a clinical, medical facility; hospitals were also social structures representing, in greater and lesser degrees, a microcosm of the world outside its walls. Moreover, film exhibition in hospitals was implemented by doctors, nurses, and patients rather than trained movie-house projectionists, thereby emphasizing film's perceived therapeutic properties. Care was taken to preselect appropriate screening materials for patient populations: "Only pictures which cheer or amuse are shown and short reels are chosen, in order that the performances may not become tiresome."[19]

This history of early media and its introduction in hospital contexts is also instructive for theories of film spectatorship and histories of exhibition practices, particularly because it complicates some of the guiding assumptions about who watches film, where, and why.[20] The exhibition of film in hospitals poses certain challenges to received ideas about film spectators. Traditional theories assume that an individual is seated in a theater, with full attention (sight and hearing intact) devoted to developing, through various psychological and affective processes, an identification with a main (usually male) character. This film spectator, assumed until the 1970s to be white and male, was also assumed to be healthy and not distracted by physical pain or spatial contexts. The idea of *hospital* film exhibition and spectatorship calls for a rethinking of what it means to watch film, and how our physical condition and the location of our spectatorship matter.

Film spectators in a hospital context might be lying in a hospital bed, propped up on pillows, watching a film with ten other people who may or may not be in hospital beds or wheelchairs, sitting or standing. As opposed to watching a film in a theater full of people sitting in comfortable positions, film spectatorship in hospitals could also be accompanied by a certain level of physical discomfort and displeasure. Whereas film spectatorship has been theorized on the basis of the pleasure and comfort of a moviegoer watching a film in a darkened theater surrounded by other presumably healthy people, film spectatorship in hospitals presupposes that the viewer will be either physically or mentally ill. Thus those individuals who are watching films while undergoing treatment or convalescing from surgery or an illness within a hospital may have a different relation to the medium than do spectators who see films in a theatrical context. The history of hospital film spectatorship makes apparent the ways that the theatrical film experience has tended to overlook the physical and mental condition of those watching (with the exception of theorizations of visual and narrative pleasure).[21] In the case of watching a film in the hospital, the corporeal experience of being a film spectator can mean very different things than what it might mean for a film spectator in a conventional theatrical context.

The Hospital Happiness Movement provides a very early example of the adaptability of film to a variety of spaces and types of spectators. Rather than the spectator going out to see films in a theater or in some other context, *the movies came to patients.* They watched in groups or as individuals, some ambulatory, some in wheelchairs, and others from their hospital beds. Theories of film spectatorship, with the exception of scholarly work on the production and reception contexts of home movies or in terms of itinerant film exhibitioners, has tended to regard the spectator as mobile—the one who goes to the movies—while the movies are located in a stationary space. But the early history of film exhibition in hospitals shows us that film was mobile, though perhaps not as mobile as radio and television broadcasts. Movies *moved* from place to place, from one non-theatrical venue to another, as historians of itinerant motion pictures have shown. Detached from a fixed theatrical exhibition space, hospital film exhibition shows a medium that can adapt to space as well as modify it.

As film entered the hospital space, it temporarily transformed the clinical site into something other than an institutional context. This transformation facilitated a new perception of the hospital as a deinstitutionalized space, where patient care also involved prescribing media for comfort and therapeutic distraction. Further, not only were films shown in places other than movie theaters, but in this particular context, as I have indicated, ideas about film spectators were revised along with ideas about what it meant to be a patient. If the ideal film spectator was understood to be in need of healing and company, then movies could be used to simultaneously respond to this need and to create a new way of experiencing the hospital as a deinstitutionalized place of individualized care and comfort.

Coinciding with revised ideas about how the modern hospital should function for its patients, the use of media such as film and radio signaled a decidedly modern response to media technology. Prescribing film and radio to its patients as a therapeutic distraction showed that hospitals were committed to providing more than medical care; they were also interested in making the hospital experience be something more than stressful or painful. This incorporation of film into the hospital routine also naturalized the place of media within this context. The therapeutic connection between media and medical care in the hospital could then be extended to the home once the patient was discharged.

By the late 1920s, some hospitals' "old institutional characters" were beginning to "give way to buildings closely resembling fine residences"; but while this may have been the case for some patients, the majority of hospitals had a long way to go before they could match such a description.[22] One agent of transformation in modernizing the hospital's institutional character came in the form of patient amenities. These included everything from carpeted private rooms, brightly painted corridors, and tasteful decorations, to the placement of fresh flowers throughout the wards and in the main circulation areas. And, of course, other significant agents of modernization came in the forms of movies and radio.

### MOTION PICTURES ARE THERAPEUTIC

Foremost among the patient-oriented turn toward the deinstitutionalized hospital was the incorporation of entertainment media. This deinstitutionalization went hand in hand with the production of the hospital as a homelike, or at least less foreboding, space. Recognizing a commercial market that was ripe for the picking, the Eastman Kodak Company's Medical Division advertised its products to hospital administrators. Although Eastman Kodak introduced a 16mm "Cine-Kodak" motion picture camera, 16mm "Kodacolor" motion picture film, and the "Kodascope" projector to the consumer market in 1923, the medical division also advertised these same products to medical institutions for educational and entertainment purposes. Indeed, Eastman made home movies practical with the introduction of 16mm Safety film, cameras, and portable projectors.[23] Eastman Kodak offered 16mm prints for rental only from various regional offices and from local camera retailers. Some of the subjects available for rental included dramas, animated cartoons, travel pictures, comedies, and educational pictures. Advertisements in *The Modern Hospital* described how easy it was to show films, noting that it was a soothing form of entertainment adaptable to a private room or crowded ward. Patients could watch their own home movies, if they had them, or other films rented from Eastman Kodak.

A 1928 advertisement reveals how Eastman Kodak's Medical Divi-

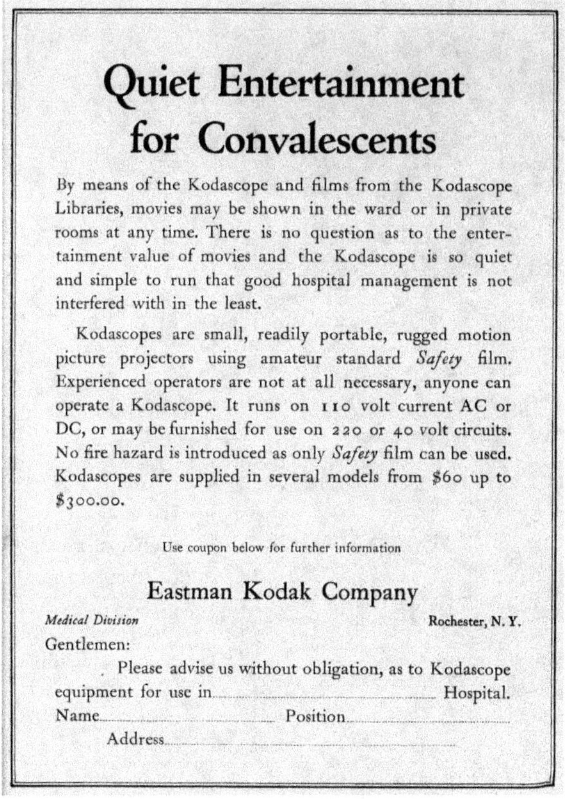

> ## Quiet Entertainment for Convalescents
>
> By means of the Kodascope and films from the Kodascope Libraries, movies may be shown in the ward or in private rooms at any time. There is no question as to the entertainment value of movies and the Kodascope is so quiet and simple to run that good hospital management is not interfered with in the least.
>
> Kodascopes are small, readily portable, rugged motion picture projectors using amateur standard *Safety* film. Experienced operators are not at all necessary, anyone can operate a Kodascope. It runs on 110 volt current AC or DC, or may be furnished for use on 220 or 40 volt circuits. No fire hazard is introduced as only *Safety* film can be used. Kodascopes are supplied in several models from $60 up to $300.00.
>
> Use coupon below for further information
>
> ### Eastman Kodak Company
>
> Medical Division      Rochester, N. Y.
> Gentlemen:
>    Please advise us without obligation, as to Kodascope equipment for use in_____ Hospital.
> Name_____ Position_____
>    Address_____

**FIGURE 1**
Motion pictures as therapeutic entertainment before television.

sion was aware of the specific needs of hospitals administrators, while also selling their products through a medicalized discourse of patient comfort and convalescence. In the advertisement "Quiet Entertainment for Convalescents," which appeared in *The Modern Hospital*, Eastman Kodak tells hospital administrators that "by means of the Kodascope and films from the Kodascope Libraries, movies may be shown in the ward or in private rooms at any time" (see figure 1).[24] The advertisement describes Kodascopes as "small, readily portable, rugged motion picture projectors using amateur standard *Safety* film," and states that "experienced operators are not at all necessary, anyone can operate a Kodascope." The ad includes a free-use coupon at the bottom to encourage administrators to try the Kodascope and the accompanying Kodak-produced films (or amateur film, perhaps shot by patients with the newly available Cine-Kodak).

Convalescent Companions     [ 33 ]

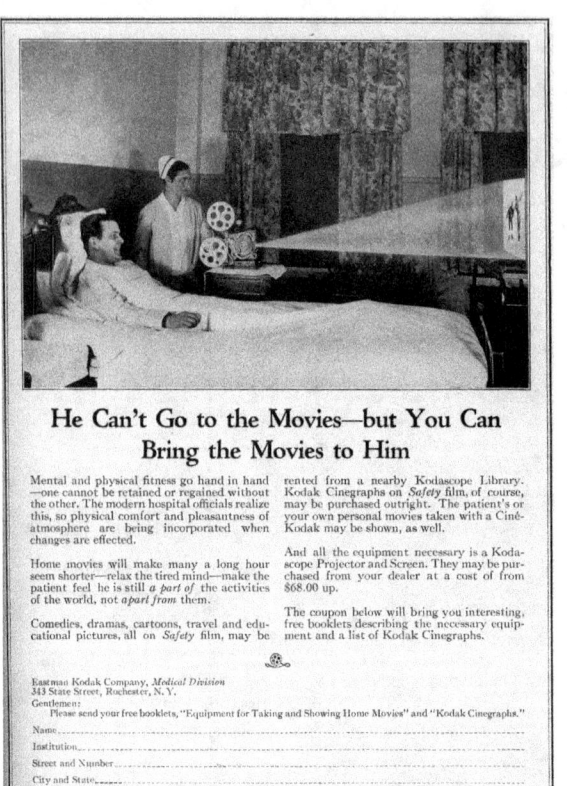

**FIGURE 2**
Motion pictures connect patients to the outside world.

In a similar way, a 1930 advertisement for Eastman's "Kodak Cinegraphs" and the portable "Kodascope Projector and Screen" includes a large black-and-white photograph of a white, male patient propped up on pillows in a hospital bed as he watches a film projected on a screen on the other side of the room. Standing next to his bed is a white, female nurse, in cap and gown, operating the portable film projector (see figure 2).[25] Below the photograph of this non-theatrical form of spectatorship, the ad directly addresses hospital administrators: "He Can't Go to the Movies—but You Can Bring the Movies to Him." Eastman Kodak encourages the use of "comedies, dramas, cartoon, travel and educational pictures, all on *Safety* film," or the projection of the patient's own home movies. At the bottom of the advertisement, Eastman Kodak includes a mail-in request coupon for two free booklets: "Equipment for Taking and Showing Home Movies" and "Kodak Cinegraphs." Through the reference to personal movies, Eastman Kodak signals how film could be used to connect home and hospital and suggests that hospitals might produce their own films to show to patients. The ad also describes film as the means through which patients could be *at home* in the hospital.

These advertisements are rich for the ways that they frame film spectatorship contrary to the conventional theatrical setting. For one thing, they show that film spectatorship may serve as a therapeutic device to "make the patient feel he is still *a part of* the activities of the world, not *apart from* them." Using the advertising discourse that also accompanied broadcast radio's installation into homes and hospitals—the idea of portability and connectivity—Eastman Kodak represents film as a mobile medium. Describing how "mental and physical fitness go hand in hand," Eastman Kodak uses therapeutic discourse to sell administrators on hospital film exhibition for private or ward patients. Additionally, this advertisement includes the possibility of a direct response from the subject of address, in this case, a hospital administrator or some other reader in charge of ordering such "amenities" for their institutions.

It was not only the Eastman Kodak Medical Division that promoted film as a means of therapeutic diversion. Even hospital personnel and administrators regarded film as "a cheap and practical solution of one of the hospital's greatest problems—how to keep the convalescent happy."[26] Throughout the 1920s, the Eastman Kodak Medical Division advertised films, film cameras, and projectors while various public organizations and associations continued to emphasize the possible negative social and moral effects of motion picture spectatorship.

For example, practically coinciding with the emergence of cinema itself, individuals loosely organized around a middle-class concern for social welfare made accusations of moral corruption against film content. From the 1897 *People v. Doris* court case involving allegations of indecency on film to the landmark 1915 *Mutual Film Corporation v. Industrial Commission of Ohio*, film had become an increasingly urgent target of reformers. During the first decade of the twentieth century, the Progressive reformers, comprising new middle-class professionals who sought to address social problems caused by phenomena associated with urbanization, industrialization, and immigration, set their sites on nickelodeons and, later, movie houses and other cheap leisure entertainments. Informed by Protestant religious ideology and bolstered by research from the newly emerging fields of sociology and psychology, the Progressives saw motion pictures as capable of informing as well as entertaining the public. But it was also the Progressives' understanding of film's capacity to corrupt through entertainment that was the biggest reason for concern. They feared that the movies, if not properly regulated, could influence spectators to engage in immoral activities and lead to all manner of vice. Indeed, it seems that the idea was to properly channel the power of motion pictures through careful monitoring practices so that the spectators could be protected against the excessive and indecent aspects of the medium. When the Supreme Court heard the appeal in the 1915 *Mutual Film Corporation* case, the justices unanimously decreed that film was not free speech and thus was not subject to protections granted other media such as newspapers. Relying on what was at the time and would later prove rather specious claims about motion pictures, the Supreme Court reaffirmed the Ohio state constitution's role in censoring film. By declaring that films were not free speech, but were instead a "business pure and simple, originated and conducted for profit, like other cheap spectacles, not intended to be regarded by the Ohio constitution . . . as part of the press of the country or as an organ of popular opinion," the Supreme Court paved the way for further organized, nationwide efforts to censor and regulate movie content.[27] One of the many consequences of this ruling was the development of "Better Films Committees" and the Hays Office of the Motion Picture Producers and Distributors of America, founded in 1922 to implement and enforce Hollywood's notorious Production Code.

The 1915 Supreme Court decision seemed to consider context a determining factor for saying that film was not a medium in the way a newspaper is, even though both are profit-driven businesses. Rather, the justices said unanimously that film had more in common with circuses and sideshows than it did with legitimate vehicles for public opinion such as newspapers and magazines. In this way, it is instructive to think about how hospital exhibition of film occurred at all, given the public concern over the potentially immoral or otherwise harmful aspects of the movies. One can see how context shapes spectatorship and meaning. Within an already hygienic venue such as a hospital, the concerns about the deleterious effects of the movies might be lessened, or moviegoing even rendered a healthy and therapeutic experience.[28] Thus, as moral debates about the role of motion pictures and society continued outside hospital walls, the use of motion pictures inside seems to have been understood very differently. This contrast between public criticism of film, and later radio, was also to be echoed in relation to the new medium of television some thirty years later.

Film and radio offered their audiences different experiences in the context of the theater, hospital, or home. Both film and radio are mass media, but in different ways. Film is a mass medium to the extent that many spectators can see the same film, but not necessarily all at the same time. Radio is a mass medium to the extent that it is broadcast from one point but reaches many listeners. Unlike film, it addresses us together and as individuals at the same time, from one place to different places. Film and radio also appeal to different senses, as the radio historian Susan Douglas has documented. But the main distinction between film and radio involves time. While spectators might see the same film, they might not see it at the same time, whereas radio listeners might be separated by space, but they can be united through time and the broadcast signal. Listeners in a hospital in midtown Manhattan might be united with their friends or family in Brooklyn or a city in upstate New York simply by tuning in to the same radio program, at the same time. Radio and television liveness makes their use in hospitals very different from the experience of film spectatorship in hospitals. The connectivity and sharing of simultaneous listening *and* viewing made available by radio and television offered listeners and viewers a sense of shared temporality that could mediate distance.

### RADIO: NEWS OF THE WELL WORLD

More than movies, broadcast radio promised to connect hospital patients to the outside world. But just as patients, staff, and administrators praised radio for its ability to bring the outside world in, it also provided a means of creating a sense of the hospital as a specific kind of social community. Radio, because of its technological specificity —the reception and amplification of sound, and the medium's use of sound recording techniques—also offered the possibility, through simultaneous listening, of connecting hospital patients to friends and family. The installation of radio gave patients the means, if only through their imaginations, to feel less confined. Radio may have been experienced as contact with the outside world, but it was also a form of contact shaped through a consensus of taste and administrative oversight.[29] As review boards regulated the films exhibited to soldiers at the front as well as in the hospital during the First World War, so did hospital administrators control the types of radio and other sound programming to which their patients had access. Audience reception was determined in no small part by what was deemed appropriate for the health and well-being of the listeners.

In contrast to film exhibition in hospitals, radio enabled hospital patients to listen, in real time, to the same songs and programs that friends and family were listening to at home. This experiential quality of radio, its perceived characteristics of immediacy and connectivity, would also be used to describe the function of television for hospital patients. Although patients were separated from friends and family, radio and television advertisers suggested, at least they could imagine that they were connected to loved ones by listening to the same radio programs, or watching the same television shows. The sense of simultaneity was specific to broadcast radio and television. Radio and television manufacturers used simultaneity and the simulation of shared time and space as a means of marketing these media to hospitals.

During the early 1920s, as radio manufacturers, broadcasters, and the federal government struggled to set the parameters of modern radio broadcasting, hospitals were among the first customers for the installation of sound amplification systems and radio sets. For example, in 1923 *Hygeia*, the consumer magazine of the American Medical Association, told readers that Beth Israel Hospital in New York provided radio for patients. Offering a "radio plug for every bed," Beth Israel utilized a central public address system to distribute radio, phonograph recordings, and hospital announcements through general loudspeakers and headsets. Three years after the radio station KDKA broadcast the 1920 national presidential election results that declared Warren G. Harding the winner, Beth Israel Hospital in New York City boasted, "Rx: One dose of radio to be taken before bedtime."[30] Framing the new medium of radio as a sedative, patients plugged their individual headsets into newly installed bedside radios in the hope that soothing music or other programs might be a "sleeping potion for some of the patients who worry and do not sleep well."[31]

Hospitals utilize various technologies of listening and sound reproduction. From physicians listening through stethoscopes to patients' bodies for signs of illness, to the use of telephone systems and other internal and external communication devices, to the introduction of recorded music and amplification systems and radio, recorded sound offers a way of condensing and collecting information as well as experience. As Jonathan Sterne keenly explains in relation to the difference between collective "technical listening" and "collective entertainment listening," radio functioned in hospitals as a means of bringing patients together and organizing temporal as well as spatial relations, while it also offered privatized experiences of both *live* and *recorded* sound.[32] The mass-market dissemination of headphones enabled several individuals to listen collectively to a phonograph or a radio. This technological and cultural development, when placed in an institutional context such as a hospital, had the effect of creating a shared sense of space while also ensuring that entertainment sound would not interrupt technical sound (the capacity for physicians to listen to one another, patients, and nurses, and for other aural communication to function, such as telephone systems). Creating a collective, shared experience of therapeutic entertainment had the potential to also revise the perception of the hospital as a deinstitutionalized space where patients were isolated from one another, and to connect them to family and friends elsewhere, if only by listening to the same radio program.

Moreover, radio as a mass medium held out certain promises and possibilities compared to other media such as film. According to Michele Hilmes, "More than any other medium, radio seemed in its early days to lend itself to association with ideas of nation, of national identity, to 'the heart and mind of America,' its 'soul.'"[33] This association with "ideas of nation" is made explicit by radio's broadcasting status as a "government-regulated extension of the public sphere."[34] As such, this gave the new medium and the "experience of 'listening in' more weight and influence than going to the movies or reading a popular magazine; its status as a semipublic institution charged with tasks of education and cultural uplift put it on par with other official institutions, such as schools, churches, and the government itself."[35] Each of these promises of unity—whether in the form of a normative English language or of the utopian ideal of uniting the nation—also had its potential problems. Yet, in ways that film could not approach, radio was experienced both as a privatized and collective phenomenon and, as in the case of hospital contexts, something that could provide a sense of comfort and familiarity to patients spatially separated from home, friends, and families.

The hospital trade publication *Hospital Management* reported in 1925 that radio had been approved for use and installed in "45 of the hospitals of the U.S. Veteran's Bureau." To put the figure into perspective and to emphasize the magnitude of the installations, this included "an approximate total of 337 loudspeakers and 7,276 headsets of earphones." The report describes the technical process for installing radio into existing structures and those under construction. Interestingly, the report notes that for different kinds of hospitals, different management and control of listening materials may be required. "Neuropsychiatric hospitals" are to use only loudspeakers; "tuberculosis and general hospitals" provide a "head set at each bed" and loudspeakers in "wards and assembly rooms."[36] The report's lack of explanation of the difference in the installation methods among hospitals suggests that mental patients may have been given less agency to control the uses of radio; it seemed they were more subject, at least potentially, to the choices of the administering staff than were other kinds of patients. It may also indicate an implicit assumption regarding the management of external stimuli for nervous patients. Although this may not have been the case, it is significant that this distinction between mental and physical illness should be reproduced through the disciplined, technical application of entertainment forms to sick bodies or sick minds. Thus, showing particular films or playing particular radio programs and music not only has an assumed therapeutic function, but also exerts an applied management of bodies and minds.

Early use of radio in a general hospital context is, apart from the industrial history, an important account of the relationship between the hospital set operator and the listeners. Although the listening material was determined to a degree, no doubt, by signal strength and the availability of stations, it was also shaped by the taste preferences of staff and patients. *Hospital Management* states that the operator was to be "advised of the patient's preferences" in selecting listening materials or programs. Yet the operator made the final decision about where to set the radio dial. The report does make a point of noting that in hospitals where headsets were available, patients could simply not listen or "plugout without interfering [in] the pleasure of others."[37] As the above description suggests, radio communication in hospitals was anything but direct, mediated as it was through each level of the transmission and reception process. Just as hospital administrators and staff matched film genre to the mental and physical conditions of patients, so did they also program listening experiences.

Recognizing the possible utility, in a different sense, of radio in hospitals, the infamous and entrepreneurial physician of questionable credibility Dr. John R. Brinkley built his own radio station, KFKB ("Kansas Folks Know Best" or "Kansas First, Kansas Best"), and began to broadcast in 1923.[38] KFKB was located adjacent to his hospital, the Brinkley Institute of Health, built in 1918. Dr. Brinkley ran the radio station and the hospital and accepted no advertising, with the exception of the promotion of his various treatments and cure-alls. KFKB featured only live music; no recorded music was played. When live music was not played, Dr. Brinkley broadcast his own lectures on healthy living. Along with these lectures, he also had a question-and-answer show focusing on common medical concerns from a wide range of listeners. His main audience, however, consisted of his current patients next door at the hospital, or those listeners likely to become patients, mostly rural farm families. His hospital in Milford also included a research laboratory and training school for nurses (especially those with expertise in caring for his particular medical specialization in male rejuvenation).[39] The story of Brinkley's innovative melding of down-home medical advice—commercialism combined with health information—with the encouragement of consumers to regard themselves as potential patients through the new medium of radio, can be seen as a precursor to more contemporary mass-media practices found in the medical marketplace. Without a doubt, Brinkley's legitimacy and relationship to patient care was questionable, but his early use of radio to create a public interested in health and accustomed to hearing messages about these medical concerns is echoed in today's medical pitchmen, perhaps most obviously in the phenomenon of direct-to-consumer drug advertising.

In a similar precursor to advertising in the contemporary medical marketplace, a 1925 article titled "Doctors Are Preferred Prospects," published in the industry trade magazine *Radio Retailing*, describes how radio sellers should focus on physicians as an obvious market for the use of "radio treatment."[40] As drugs "cure the body," so "radio cures the mind on which the body is dependent."[41] Indeed, physicians prompted by their own experience with radio and by sellers' suggestions saw radio as yet another necessary electrical device (like the X-ray) in treating their patients. *Radio Retailing* quotes a physician who sees a direct connection between patient recovery and radio listening:

> Keeping the patient contented, and his mind at ease and free from worry over his condition is one of the chief problems a doctor must face. . . . A radio set puts him in the right mental attitude with the least effort. Listening to a

talk or a concert, he forgets himself and his illness. His mind is cured and the recovery of his body is thus materially aided. It is the psychological effect of radio on the patient's mind that makes it such a wonderful aid to recovery. If a patient lacks the will to live or to recover, he is frequently doomed beforehand. But if he hears continually the good things that are coming over the air, although subconsciously perhaps, he will, nevertheless, acquire first the desire, then the determination, to go on living.[42]

This passage from *Radio Retailing* underscores the idea that radio can be, in certain doses and under certain conditions, a type of aural therapy. Not limited to radio sellers and manufacturers, medical professionals promoted the therapeutic value of mass media as well. Even more than human contact or the power of modern medicine, the physician quoted in the passage above grants radio the abilities to heal first the mind, then the body, of patients who may lack "the will to live or to recover." The implicit assumption is that radio voices and, as we saw with the case of film, moving images are therapeutic by virtue of their ability to temporarily distract patients from their pain and discomfort. In so doing, the incorporation of therapeutic media within the hospital allows the medical space to be experienced in a different way. As I argue throughout the book, one of the consequences of this turn to patient entertainment and comfort is the deinstitutionalization of the built environment of the hospital. If hospitals could be re-imagined as spaces where patient solace and comfort are just as important as medical treatment—indeed if media become therapeutic treatments—then hospitals may be experienced as places where patients feel they could not only potentially be cured, but be cared for as well.

Framed as a philanthropic gesture, radio dealers were encouraged to sell radio to institutions as a form of institutional citizenship. Advertisements and articles in trade retailer publications emphasized ways to appeal to hospital administrators' and physicians' sense of benevolence and to patient need by incorporating radio into hospitals and doctors' offices. Hospitals could represent themselves as concerned institutional citizens through their obvious incorporation of media. The use of radio in hospitals also helped to reconnect isolated patients to important events happening in their lives outside hospital walls, emphasizing their continued participation in the healthy world. *Radio Retailing* promoted to wholesale and retail radio sellers the idea that, especially for "hospitals, homes, sanitariums, and charitable institutions of all kinds," radio was a medium of transport, connection, and transformation. For veterans of the First World War at military hospitals, the New York State Association for the Blind, or any other hospital, radio music and programs "while away the weary, bedridden hours" or help the blind to "visualize the world."[43]

Contrary to film and television, individual radio sets in *The Modern Hospital* were advertised less often than were sound amplification and transmission systems. By 1930 the Radio Receptor Co. proclaimed the virtues of its Powerizer Sound Systems through an illustrated advertisement that featured male patients listening to a boxing match.[44] Although the male listeners are depicted sitting together, each of them wears a blanket and a set of headphones. The Powerizer Sound Systems, licensed by the Radio Corporation of America and Associated Companies, tells hospital administrators that enabling "red-blooded men about ready to be discharged from a hospital" to listen to a "prize fight, a ball game or any other form of program that would cause a temperature in the case of a neurotic," would surely speed along their recoveries. Given the hearty nature of masculinity, apparently, administrators need not worry about the male patients being easily overwhelmed by negative emotions (as might befall a listener with less mental stamina). This inherent strength of red-blooded men is also emphasized through the name of the product, which suggests a masculinization of radio listening, as "real" men enjoy sports such as prize fighting and baseball.

In a 1931 advertisement titled "And Bolster Up His Spirits with Music," Western Electric also emphasizes that music speeds patient recovery (see figure 3). The ad displays a male patient lying in bed as he listens to music through a headset. The written text below the image describes how, with the addition of the Western Electric Public Address and Music Reproducing System, "music helps patients to pass pleasantly hours of recuperation that would otherwise drag. And music is a medicine . . ."[45] This advertisement is interesting for the way that it represents not only the product, but also a commonsensical view of the nature of the hospital experience from the patient's perspective. Understood as a drab place where time lingers, the hospital is represented as the antithesis of a happy time. The ad also raises the question of the *experience* of healing. Usually understood as the very embodiment of passivity, this advertisement seems to recognize that patients are at least mentally active and that healing is a process. The vision of the patient as active, to an extent, in his or her own healing process will be key to understanding how

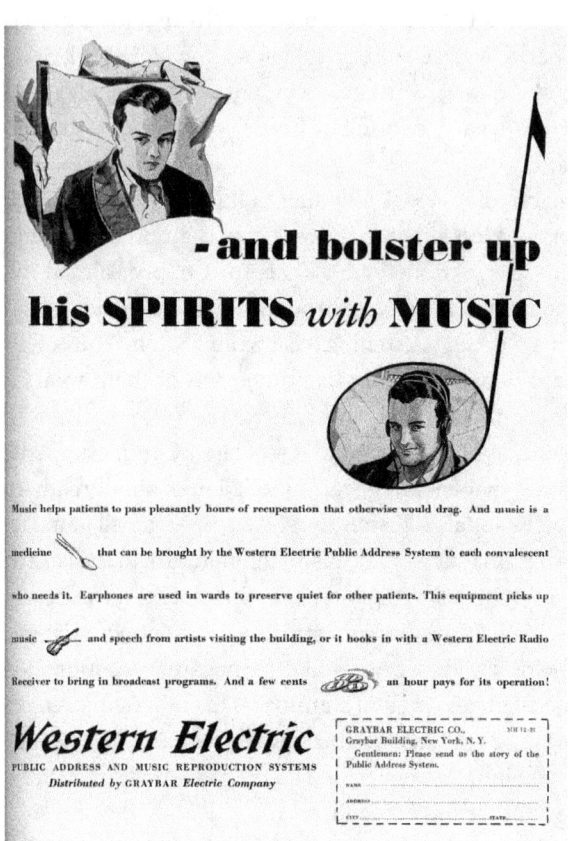

FIGURE 3
Recuperative and privatized listening—radio in hospitals.

prescription drug advertisements, more than seventy years later, function in their address to active consumer-patients.

Children also, apparently, benefit from radio's healing soundtrack, as an August 1935 Western Electric advertisement from *Hospital Management* suggests.[46] Describing Western Electric as the maker of "public address and program distribution services," the advertisement features a young white girl wearing a headset while sitting upright in a white metal bed. Wearing a clean, white nightgown and a bright smile, the little girl looks directly into the camera. With the title "Is Yours a Cheerful Hospital?," the advertisement addresses hospital administrators. The reply, "Where MUSIC speeds up recovery," appears right above a nightstand that displays a medicine bottle, glass of water, and spoon. Implying that music can be medicine, and good, economical medicine at that, Western Electric tells administrators, "Hospitals that are Western Electric equipped make their patients more cheerful than other hospitals do." Western Electric suggests that the goal of such musical entertainment systems is patient cheer and satisfaction. These advertisements tend to feature the reception or consumption end of the process, with virtually all images focusing on the patients. This emphasizes that what manufacturers are concentrating on is not *distribution* as much as *reception* (the effects that radio will have on patients as the ideal receivers).

Another element that stands out in these advertisements for hospital film, radio, and later television systems, is the way nurses are routinely represented as the operators of these machines. In fact, nurses were depicted as the ideal managers of all hospital communication systems. Whether in the form of a nurse-call system, in the operation of radio sets, or as film projectionists, nurses were shown as the obvious matrons (all the nurses featured in articles and advertisements are female) of communication and entertainment technologies. By the early 1950s, the nurse call and the controls for radio and television would be integrated into a single remote control device. This device would also include a small speaker through which the patient could hear the radio, television, and nurse. As a more fully developed version of the early radio pillow, these remote devices would replace bulky headsets as the preferred sound transmission and reception system.[47]

The dissemination of radio followed the adoption of communication or signaling systems. During the same time that hospitals were installing individual radio sets for use in group or ward areas, they were also wiring buildings for voice-sound amplification systems. The mid-to-late 1920s saw a marked increase in advertisements for signal-phone systems and articles discussing the new communication demands placed on nurses and hospital staff. Advertisements for signaling systems, such as one published in 1925 in *Hospital Management* for the Chicago Silent Call Signal System, manufactured by the Chicago Signal Co., emphasized the immediacy of contact between patient and nurse (see figure 4).[48] Featuring an illustration of a female patient and her visitor, the advertisement emphasizes the efficiency and convenience of signal systems, connecting patients to nurses. In an accompanying advertisement, again from the Chicago Signal Co., the illustration shows a nurse trying "to beat Death itself to the sickbed," sprinting down the hall with the Grim Reaper hot on her heels. The quicker a patient can communicate with a nurse, the better for both. Most often in advertisements for nurse-

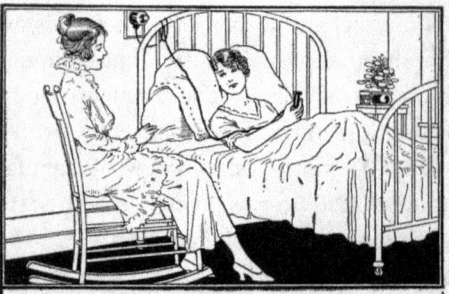

FIGURE 4
Silent signaling—the Chicago Signal Co.

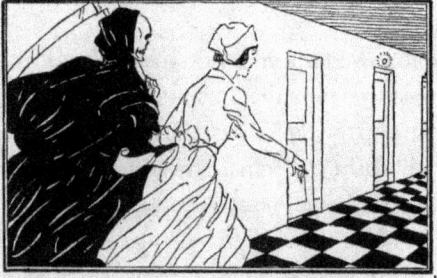

FIGURE 5
Beating death through efficient and rapid nurse labor—the Chicago Signal Co.

call or signal systems, it was the nurses' attention that was represented as the most significant in terms of patient care (see figure 5).[49] In both of the signal system advertisements, the connection between patient and nurse is dependent upon technological immediacy and reliability. While communities and households across the country were experiencing the pleasures and possibilities of radio as a *broadcast* medium, hospitals were some of the earliest adopters of various kinds of point-to-point communication and mass media technologies—from telephones and hospital-switchboard nurse-call signaling systems, to film, radio, and television.

A 1929 advertisement in *The Modern Hospital* for the Dictograph Production Company promises to add "a unique telephonic contact between patient and nurse made possible by the super-sensitive Dictograph microphone and soft speaker."[50] In addition to existing signaling systems—such as door lamps and corridor lamps, which acted as codes to alert nurses and doctors to particular patient needs—voice or sound systems such as that provided by Dictograph Production offered instant communication. As hospitals grew in size, and nurses had to travel farther and farther to care for patients, these new systems offered better service to patients and increased efficiency for nurses' labor. Both of these signaling systems were selling certainty of communication, following in a long historical trajectory that understood technologies of communication, from the telegraph to the television, as capable of sending and receiving signals with a fidelity and speed that had not existed before. While the precision of communication was more of an ideal, a way of selling communication systems such as the Dictograph or radio, it nonetheless was a commodity that hospitals, because of their specific need to provide for the efficient and rapid transmission of messages, would buy. Hospitals could, in turn, promote their institutions as having not only state-of-the-art medical capabilities but also cutting-edge communication systems that were reliable and necessary for saving lives. Communication systems also produced a sense that nurses, and potentially doctors, could be everywhere all at once, a comforting idea for patients. The ads suggest that speed and efficiency can conquer space and time.

These advertisements speak to how the presence of media marketing discourses and specific practices can influence the actual material history of watching and listening in the hospital environment. As film, radio, and television entered the hospital space, the patient was constructed as a specific kind of spectator, listener, or viewer who experienced media differently. In the context of a hospital, film spectatorship may be experienced as a connection to the outside world and as a way of seeing the hospital as a space of patient-oriented comfort. While surely contributing to patient ease and playing a key role in deinstitutionalizing the hospital space, media technologies such as film and radio also joined other components of the modern hospital to create a sense of connection between the hospital and home. From the late 1910s through the 1930s, hospitals in the United States began to radically reimagine the ways that the public perceived them. In professional publications such as *The Modern Hospital*, aimed at hospital administrators, articles instructed their readers about how interior design, as well as patient amenities, could not only increase their revenue, but also make the hospital seem less like a clinical institution and more like a familiar home. As part of this process of deinstitutionalization, new mass entertainment media such as film and radio created new possibilities for patient therapeutic care and comfort. Treating the patient included doses of therapeutic entertainment as well as medical care. Indeed, movies became medicine, as the Hospital Happiness Movement made clear.

Film and radio, in making their entrance into hospital spaces, transformed those spaces through their mere presence. Considered at first to be unwelcome guests by hospital staff, they became accepted features of hospitals once administrators realized how film and radio might function to increase patients' senses of well-being and comfort. Film and radio literally made space for the new medium of television by showing the ways that mass media could provide a sense of connection to the outside world—namely, to friends and family beyond the hospital walls. Mass media could also promote active mental engagement through the pleasures of watching one's favorite film or through collective, shared listening to a live sporting event or concert. For patients otherwise limited in their physical capacities, film, radio, and, as will be examined in the following two chapters, television, offered them the opportunity to be transported, if only in a figurative and imaginative sense, to other places and other, perhaps more pleasurable experiences.

## Television Goes to the Modern Hospital

The introduction of various forms of entertainment also coincided with hospitals' efforts at institutional transformation (or at least the transformation of how hospitals were regarded by the public). Motion pictures and other media need to be understood as part of this attitudinal shift in relation to twentieth-century medical care and the rise of health care consumerism. In order for hospitals to attract patients, the institutions needed to have a less daunting image. Before it was possible to imagine themselves as health consumers, people had to be taught to think of hospitals and clinics in new ways. Primed by the introduction of film and radio decades earlier, I argue that television has been the principal means by which this change in perception has come about.[1] Film and radio facilitated structural and perceptual shifts not only in the ways hospitals represented themselves to patients as deinstitutionalized spaces of medical care, but they also began a process of naturalizing linkages among media, medicine, and patients. The consequences of this naturalization can be seen, in an obvious way, through the structural placement of television in hospitals as well as in the increasingly health-oriented programming offered in the form of entertainment and education.

While the story of television's installation into homes in the United States during the post–Second World War years has been well documented, less attention has been paid to how television came to be a commonplace fixture in hospitals. Television was first admitted into hospitals in 1947 as a medium of instruction for medical students and nursing staff, and just a few years later, in 1950, as a form of therapeutic entertainment for patients. But television's entry into hospitals from the late 1940s through the 1960s was accompanied by innovations in hospital architecture that emphasized the role of spatial design in improving a patient's overall experience of hospitalization.

If the introduction of television into hospitals functioned as a means of humanizing health care institutions, then what were the implicit assumptions that accompanied its installation? What roles did devices such as television—as well as aspects of interior design, architectural practices, and aesthetics—serve in the deinstitutionalization of modern hospitals? Drawing both from scholarly studies of television's installation in homes in the United States and examinations of television as a form of public amusement in places outside non-institutional domestic residences, this chapter attends to the various ways that television was incorporated into hospitals.[2] Far from tangential, television has been central to the development and transformation of the hospital and the rise of modern health consumerism in the United States. Perhaps not surprisingly, given that hospitals have provided one of the most familiar contexts for dramatic programming, the bulk of television scholarship has taken the form of close readings of various doctor dramas, while the specificity of television *in* hospitals has remained unexplored. The initial entrance of television into this space changed its status from luxurious amenity to standard equipment. As television has become omnipresent in many different non-domestic settings over the past few decades—a common and expected feature in shopping malls, on airplanes, and in automobiles—it has also become standard in health care settings.

Yet television also can serve as a prism through which we can see larger issues regarding health and the medical industry. By examining its material history in the hospital, we can also better understand how television functions elsewhere in non-medical settings to provide us with information about our daily lives. Through the microcosm of television, we can learn about how the macrocosm of hospitals and medicalization function to produce us as consumer-patients. Reviewing the architectural history of television's placement in hospitals allows us to analyze the practical considerations of how the medium was incorporated into the hospital and how it has continued to function as a medicalizing discourse in contemporary culture. Television's materiality is also discursive in that it facilitates a particular production of medical institutions and medicalized subjects. Given this, I examine the discourses and architectural innovations that facilitated television's arrival, and the conditions for its reception, in the institutional context of the modern, postwar hospital in the United States.

Mapping television's physical installation in hospitals involves sifting through several different layers of archival materials, including architectural plans and illustrations, editorials in trade publications such as *The Modern Hospital* and *Hospitals* (the publication of the American Hospital Association), and advertisements, which I will examine in detail in the following chapter. As pieces of historical evidence in their own right, they offer ways of making sense of how television came to be an accepted piece of equipment in the modern hospital. Although popular magazines offered "pictorial displays of television sets in domestic settings," advertisements in *The Modern Hospital* suggested to hospital administrators (mostly men) and other hospital workers (including nurses and dieticians, mostly women) ways to integrate television into this institutional space.[3] Television in patient rooms was used as a way of contributing to and facilitating a familiar sense of home in a place that was, in some ways, strange and unfamiliar. Hospitals, particularly in the 1960s, grew larger and larger; administrators tried to create a sense of intimacy in an increasingly overwhelming space. Television, along with experiments in interior design, became a means of injecting humanism and familiarity into these contexts.

Both in terms of aiding the fiscal state of hospitals and the physical condition of patients, television manufacturers encouraged hospital administrators to make television more than a mere amenity. Advertisers gave administrators various ways to use television in hospitals. Through promotional examples, manufacturers explained how television—through closed-circuit educational programs, patient surveillance, and diversion or entertainment—could indeed go hand in hand with the self-described mission of the modern mega-hospital.[4] Administrators, in turn, responded to advertisers' suggestions and patients' demands for incorporating television into the overall mission of mid-century hospitals. Part of that mission included the construction of carefully crafted and managed public images that, as the hospital historian Rosemary Stevens observes, represented modern hospitals as "having something valuable to sell: surgery, glamour, expertise, healthy babies."[5] In a competitive medical marketplace, hospitals used television, at least initially, to attract middle-class and other patients who had the ability to pay for private rooms and medical procedures. Thus modern hospitals tended to display a contradictory vision of health care institutions: one that represented all that was technologically sophisticated, or most unlike home, combined with a comforting, homelike structure.

Spigel analyzes women's decorating magazines from the 1950s as discursive sites that represent a history of television's installation in the private home. But *professional* or trade hospital magazines, such as *The Modern Hospital*, from that same time tell an equally rich story about television's circulation and reception in spaces outside the home. Asked to manage their hospitals as housewives manage efficient, modern homes, hospital administrators turned to *The Modern Hospital* for advice on a variety of issues and topics. Divided into generic categories based on the hospital's division of labor, each issue of the magazine highlighted a "Hospital of the Month." Presented as ideals, these Hospitals of the Month served as models for administrators or other decision-making personnel to follow in constructing new hospitals or in renovating existing ones. From industry-friendly analyses of the impact of new federal Medicare legislation to recipes for hospital kitchens, the magazine addressed hospital administrators as its primary audience. These texts told managers and administrators how to incorporate television into patient rooms and other hospital areas.

Replete with architectural plans for hospital renovation and advice about such things as noise reduction for clamorous hallways, *The Modern Hospital* served as a professional version of popular home-design magazines. Although Spigel's analysis of such magazines focuses on female consumers, *The Modern Hospital* was a trade publication that addressed both male (administrators) and female (nurses, dieticians) readers. But its status as a limited-circulation, professional magazine distinguished it from mass-circulation magazines such as *Ladies' Home Journal* or *American Home*. Nonetheless, *The Modern Hospital*, like popular home-focused magazines, framed its representation of the institution through the lens of domesticity (with explicitly gendered labor categories). The magazine's advertisements and feature articles address a market that is defined by its *institutional*, rather than *individual*, buying power.

This trade magazine also provided a forum for nationwide debates about contemporary social issues, such as the desegregation of hospitals and the role of administrators in ensuring that their hospitals met new hiring standards and policies for non-discriminatory patient care. *The*

*Modern Hospital* published condensed reports regarding the changing relationship between the hospital industry and the federal government through the implementation of Great Society Programs such as the Civil Rights Act of 1964 and the creation of the Medicare system in 1965. Amid some of the most substantial shifts ever to occur in the health care industry in the United States, television was introduced as the prescription for ailing institutions. Manufacturers represented television as having the capacity to evoke a sense of home and familiarity for patients who found themselves surrounded by strangers in an unfamiliar context. For homesick patients, television viewing provided just the cure. Watching their favorite television programs in a potentially distressing context may have enabled viewers to feel more at home in the hospital. Additionally, the reliability and performance offered by the sets signified the scientific and technical sophistication of the institution.

But television's entrance into the hospital was not unencumbered. Before television could become part of the daily operation of hospitals, administrators had to decide where it would go, how it would be installed, and who would administer it to whom. Typical managerial questions, no doubt, but strategic ones as well. In economic and structural senses, television had to be made to fit into established work patterns and into certain hospital protocols regarding patient care, surveillance, and visitations from family and friends. Television's initial entrance into the hospital was pragmatic to the extent that it not only provided a way to help patients pass time, but it also facilitated surveillance and monitoring. Thus television combined patient entertainment with closed-circuit programming and patient surveillance systems. From patient visitations via television to do-it-yourself, nurse-produced educational programs for inpatients, television integrated various communication technologies into one overall system. Usually administered and controlled by female nurses, hospital television was not limited to patients watching broadcast programs in their private or semiprivate rooms. Collecting all these functions in one apparatus, television became an essential piece of medical and entertainment technology.

### MEGA-HOSPITALS AND TELEVISION: MACHINES FOR HEALING

While postwar, middle-class consumers were busy installing their sets in suburban homes, television was becoming an ordinary part of the modern hospital. Television was the perfect prescription for hospitals after the Second World War. It called attention to hospitals as the embodiment of technological sophistication and injected elements of comfort and familiarity into an increasingly intimidating material structure. Whether in houses of tomorrow or hospitals of the future, television's presence signaled the extent to which they were to be understood as, respectively, "machines for living" and "machines for healing."[6]

As the architectural historian Annmarie Adams observes in *Medicine by Design*, the history of any hospital always tells more than simply the story of a building's design and construction. As with any other building, its history is both explicit, through visible detail, aesthetic style, and function, and implicit in other features, such as the placement of patient rooms, the arrangement of nurses' stations, and the display of high-tech machines. In other words, hospitals, and other kinds of structures, can provide significant information about the role of health and healing through rather mundane objects and features—such as, in this case, the placement of television for patient entertainment. In this respect, I support Adams and other architectural historians in arguing for a consideration of the specific ways that hospitals can serve as repositories of cultural and medical records.[7]

Adams's study of the design and construction of the Royal Victoria Hospital in Montreal is one of the few analyses in the field of architecture to move beyond an examination of architectural style, form, or function to embrace the social and cultural organization of space. It also emphasizes how architectural design engages with and shapes those individuals who use the space: doctors, nurses, patients, visitors, and support staff. One of the key aspects of Adams's case study that is most relevant for understanding hospitals as social institutions is that she shares the sense that there is more than a structural connection between spaces and use of space. As she observes, "Linking architectural spaces to everyday hospital activities such as meal preparation and waiting to see a doctor is an equally important aspect.... As institutions that never close and are thus in constant motion, hospitals are ideal buildings in which to study use."[8] Adams adds that she has yet to find a document that describes the preferred movements of the building's users, but that the Royal Victoria did and continues to incorporate existing social and cultural categories of race, gender, and class into its material, spatial organization. Depending on one's race, class, or gender, for example, patients and staff "moved through the hospital in fundamentally different ways."[9]

Along with her analysis of design plans and blueprints for the Royal Victoria Hospital, Adams is keenly interested in the material culture of hospital machines, furnishings, and the things that have taken shape along with modern medicine in institutional contexts. She regards hospitals as historical and constantly changing collections of artifacts whose content suggests much about the aesthetic, scientific, and medical aspects of daily life within such spaces. As Adams explains, "A substantial part of approaching hospitals as artifacts of material culture is taking a closer look at the stuff inside them (furniture, finishes, technologies, everything) than is usually the case in architectural history. The design and placement of radiators, blanket warmers, elevators, acoustical insulation, and bedside tables serve as evidence in this story of the sometimes tense, always interesting relationship of architecture and medicine."[10]

Following Adams, the placement of television in the modern hospital —as both a furnishing and a medical device—tells us as much about the medium as it does about the nature of the structures in which it "lives." Further, as the media and cultural studies theorist Lawrence Grossberg explains, the nature and function of the medium itself changes depending on where it is situated:

> The very force and impact of any medium changes significantly as it is moved from one context to another (a bar, a theatre, the living room, the bedroom, the beach, a rock concert . . . ). Each medium is then a mobile term taking shape as it situates itself . . . within the rest of our lives. . . . The text is located, not only intertextually, but in a range of apparatuses as well. . . . Thus, one rarely just listens to the radio, watches TV, or even goes to the movies—one is studying, dating, driving somewhere else, etc.[11]

Grossberg encourages the analysis of the ways that television may be integrated into daily routines as well as the ways that it, and other media, might interrupt other practices. As with radio, television was integrated into hospital routines while it also changed how hospitals functioned. What's more, the integration and interruption of certain devices affect not only the people maneuvering in that space, but also the nature of the space itself—even a mega-hospital.

Two typical and ubiquitous mid-twentieth-century hospital building designs in the United States were the vertical monobloc and the horizontal pavilion style. These structures towered above city skylines like "obtrusive alien bulks" or "spread over a series of city blocks like an unruly plate of spaghetti."[12] Hospitals in this style are noteworthy for their distinct lack of ornamentation and huge expanses of steel and glass. Frequently defining them by such terms as *inflexible, rigid, mechanistic*, and *flat-chested*, architectural critics have generally held great contempt for these mid-century utilitarian structures.[13]

The apparent uniformity in postwar urban hospitals needs to be understood in terms of the federal government's involvement in financing hospital construction. Part of the standardization of design was based on economic and regulatory constraints. This is not to say that economic considerations determined, in any explicit way, hospital design. Rather, it is to call attention to the legislative and economic context within which modern health care was delivered to patients. The standardization of care that was the impetus for the 1946 Hospital Survey and Reconstruction Act, commonly referred to as the Hill-Burton Act, was to be instrumental in health care architecture for decades to come. The Hill-Burton Act "offered federal assistance to state funding for renovating or building new hospitals and health centers in areas of need, including rural communities and towns with no or dilapidated pre-existing facilities."[14] One of the other stopgap measures that hospital administrators had at their disposal, a means of further humanizing or deinstitutionalizing the hospital, was *television*. Indeed, television arrived in hospitals in the United States at the same time that the standards set forth by the Hill-Burton Act were materializing, and just a few years before the passage of both the Civil Rights Act of 1964 and the Medicare legislation of 1965.

## HUMANIZING THROUGH DESIGN

After the allocation of federal funds through the Hill-Burton Act, design decisions were generally characterized by pragmatism, as patient rooms had to be arranged in a way that optimized visual surveillance. To this end, television was also used as a closed-circuit patient monitoring device that extended the nurse's watchful eye. In urban contexts, nature, or the exterior, was often brought inside the hospital with elaborate atriums and interior gardens.[15] Throughout the 1950s and 1960s, *The Modern Hospital* documented the shifts and battles in hospital design aesthetics with monthly features displaying the Hospital of the Month, usually newly constructed in a suburban area, and several other hospitals that had undertaken renovation. Located most often in urban centers, these renovated hospitals stand in marked contrast to their suburban counterparts. Rarely the object of critical architectural acclaim, hospitals have never garnered as much design prestige as, for instance, domestic or corporate built environments. Nonetheless, there was a wide and varied discussion about the ways that good design could mediate the less appealing aspects of the modern mega-hospital. With feature articles written by such noted architects as Richard J. Neutra and Frank Lloyd Wright (although neither of them actually designed a hospital), *The Modern Hospital* gave hospital administrators and other architects suggestions about how they could "inject comprehensibility and hence humanism into the modern machine hospital."[16]

For example, emphasizing the transactional aspect of our relation to buildings, Neutra challenged administrators and architects to revise the form-follows-function dictum to embrace a patient-centered approach to design. In a 1960 article titled "What Architects Should Know about Patients," Neutra observed that the form and shape of a "hospital can be formidable, repellent, frightening, or it can be hope- and confidence-inspiring and warm." Recognizing that, along with nurses and physicians, architects "too must develop the capacity to be 'patient-centered' and humane," Neutra suggests that patient experiences of hospitalization are shaped by a variety of "biophysical impacts like acoustic reverberations, glare, color, visual space itself, discomfort of positioning, problems of posture, or circulation phenomena caused by a contour bed or chair, thermal considerations—all are scrutable on different levels." Neutra says that "the designer of the human setting is, in fact, engaged in applied physiology" just as surely as is the physician. In other words, the material process of design can play a part in the performance of therapy. Interestingly, Neutra identifies what he calls optical confinement as one of the issues that designers of hospitals have to address. If the patient is "bedridden or unfree to change" his or her surroundings, this condition could exacerbate a sense of optical confinement, which would then produce an increased feeling of helplessness or entrapment.[17] Although Neutra endorses views of nature or art (representational, not abstract) as restorative solutions to the problem of optical confinement, television may also be understood as a means of combating this situation.[18]

As a response to the mechanization of patient accommodations, hospital administrators began to focus on how to make a less institutional, less clinical room. The closets, dressers, and other interior components had literally become fixed in place. As a means of addressing the uniformity and stationary aspects of patient rooms, hospital administrators began to be interested in furnishings and interior details that conveyed a less rigid sense of the space. In response, the equipment and furnishings, "once machine-like in appearance," began to take on "a softer, quasi-residential look, with many items designed to be relocated, concealed, or dismantled when not in use."[19]

If in hospitals the nurses' station serves as a centralized communication point, then the design of patient rooms has focused on the centrality of the bed.[20] Throughout the 1950s and 1960s, the patient bed began to replace the nurses' station as a space-age command center in miniature, incorporating not only the means of raising or lowering the angle of repose, but of controlling the television and nurse-call systems.[21] Second to the patient bed, the other most significant design feature of patient rooms is the window. In fact, the concept of "windowness" emphasized the potential therapeutic features of a patient's ability to see something other than medical equipment or the facing wall.[22] Yet simply having a window in a patient's room is no guarantee that the patient will be able to see through it (the back of the bed may be against the window). Moreover, at night the window becomes a mirror reflecting the interior of the room. The window view is dependent on a variety of factors, not the least of which includes the patient's own ability to see. The view through the window is, then, never an obvious one, yet research consistently has shown that patient recovery time has a correspondence with whether patients have access to windows and natural light.

Like the window, television has promised to offer its viewers a vision of the exterior world. In its introduction to consumers in the United States, as Spigel has shown, television was described as a "window on the world."[23] Offering exterior visions to confined patients, windows show the promise of an exterior life, a view of somewhere else, of life happening elsewhere even if it is not one's own. As with windowness, television also promises to take viewers beyond the confines of their dens or hospital rooms. While the window and television both frame a preselected vision of exteriority for their viewers, however, television's scale is wider. That is, even though one may not have a window with a view, the television always offers a vision of an elsewhere, even if that other place may only be a room down the hall.[24]

With respect to the relationship between therapeutic views and hospital stays, during the 1970s and 1980s the behavioral psychologist

Roger S. Ulrich conducted research at hospitals in Sweden and England, both countries with national health care systems, to investigate the relationship between positive patient outcomes and the ways that health care facilities incorporated nature (or views of nature) into their architectural designs. Ulrich found a correlation between positive patient outcomes and shortened patient hospital stays to whether patients had window views of nature and natural light, as opposed to views of the side of a brick building. Since publishing this research, Ulrich has gone on to study health care systems in Italy and Japan as well as in the United States, and he is a leading expert on the role that "supportive design" can play in health care facilities.[25] While it is not conventionally understood as part of supportive design, I maintain that television can function as a substitute window on the world and provide psychological support for patients.[26]

According to Ulrich, this theory argues that architects and designers should have as their goal the promotion of "wellness by creating physical surroundings that are 'psychologically supportive.'" "Psychologically supportive" facilities would maximize "patients' coping with the major stress accompanying illness."[27] Although this may at first sound like a philosophical component of the New Age movement, Ulrich is advocating a dynamic relationship between individuals and the spaces where they experience their daily lives. The theory of supportive design recognizes that so-called hard designs (design contexts that actually foster feelings of disorientation, anxiety, delirium, or boredom) actually contribute to sickness. Central to Ulrich's theory of architecturally supportive design is the concept of stress. Television, film, and radio have key roles to play regarding patient stress and the effects of supportive design. In this sense, I argue that television and other media that are used therapeutically could be considered elements of institutional supportive design even if they are technologies, not components of nature. Further, Ulrich has suggested that hospital designers and architects can do many things to facilitate wellness and reduce stress for patients. Even though Ulrich's research was based on studies he conducted in Europe, England, and Japan, it is just as meaningful for hospital and health care sites in the United States. Ulrich's work also demonstrates how other medical systems take a wide view of health care, one that encompasses not only "what is done to a patient, but also the patient's overall experience of the therapeutic and clinical space and its relation to successful treatment outcomes."[28]

Ulrich's theory of supportive design prescribes three ways that health care facilities may reduce patient stress. First, "health facilities should *not* raise obstacles to coping with stress, contain features that are in themselves stressors, and thereby add to the total burden of illness." Second, "health care environments should be designed to facilitate access or exposure to physical features and social situations that have stress reducing influences." Third, health facilities need to include in this formulation "patients, visitors and health care staff."[29] Apparent from Ulrich's to-do list for health facilities is the subjective nature of the goals. That is, what one patient or visitor to a health facility may experience as stress, another may experience as relaxing (or at least not stressful). Moreover, his goals tend to collapse the distinction between different types of health facilities. Do patients, visitors, or health workers expect different kinds of experiences from outpatient clinics and than they do from inpatient hospitals? Do maternity patients expect one kind of experience from hospital stays and cancer patients another?

Before further discussing television's role as a component of supportive design, however, it is necessary to emphasize that, according to Ulrich, such theories should ultimately produce three things for patients, visitors, and workers: "a sense of control with respect to physical-social surroundings; access to social support; and access to positive distractions in physical surroundings."[30] How might television provoke or mitigate a loss of control, offer a sense of connection between hospital and home, or enhance feelings of either separation or isolation?[31] Examining the discourses about the relationship between hospitals, patients, and television not only enables us to understand more about the function of television in such spaces, it also tells us about which kinds of experiences institutions would prefer their patients have.

### CONTROL OR AUTONOMY

Ulrich observes that illness "confronts patients with a number of challenges or problems that are quite stressful in part because they are uncontrollable," and observes that these feelings may be exacerbated by health facilities "that are often, for instance, noisy, confusing from the standpoint of wayfinding, invade privacy, and prevent personal control over lighting and temperature."[32] Supportive design implements strategies that enhance patients' sense of control and avoids strategies that reduce this sense. Although this may seem obvious, it is not surprising that, in terms of the relation between design and building cost, these important considerations are relegated to afterthoughts (if considered at all).[33] Along with allowing for "visual privacy for gown-clad patients in an imaging area," the second way that health facilities may best foster a sense of control for their patients is, according to Ulrich, to provide "controllable televisions in patient rooms and visitor areas."[34] Patient loss of control is increased by a lack of privacy and autonomy. Television, in this case, operates as a kind of register for the extent to which health facilities enact or deny supportive design tenets. Interestingly, it is not television per se that fosters a sense of losing control; rather, the viewers' loss of control over the conditions of reception is the source of the problem.

The notion of control has had a long history in television studies. From theories regarding the passive viewer mesmerized by the control of the television to ethnographic analyses of the gendering of the remote control device, the idea of control is central to the ways that scholars and mainstream media critics have discussed television.[35] Specifically, television viewers have been defined, in both popular and some academic accounts, as passive dupes, powerless in front of the mesmerizing screen. Fixated on the images and sounds emanating from the "boob tube," television viewers—particularly women and children—have been represented as immobilized couch potatoes or victims of the "telebug-eye."[36] This conception of the television viewer as the passive receptacle has been thoroughly critiqued by a wide range of television and mass media studies, particularly ethnographic research or reception studies. These studies take as their starting point that viewers are active, not passive, in their encounters with television. But this notion of the powerless viewer is tenacious and still shapes many current ways of conceptualizing, for example, the differences between computer users and "mere" television viewers.

It is important to observe under which conditions television viewing may be considered not only acceptable but also appropriate and encouraged. Anecdotal evidence underscores the acceptability of television viewing in places where nothing else is presumed to be going on, or in places where people have nothing better to do (i.e., in waiting areas or transitional spaces).[37] It is common to hear people rationalize their daytime television viewing by saying, "I started watching that show when I was in the hospital," or "when I was sick," or "when I was laid off from my daytime job." What such declarations underscore is a continuing need to explain television viewing. Apparently, viewing is justified only through certain circumstances (e.g., hospitalization, illness, loss of employment).

## THERAPEUTIC AND ECONOMIC VALUE OF PRIVATE ENTERTAINMENT

Hospitalization may involve prolonged periods of time in which patients are separated from friends, family, and home—anything that is familiar and part of his or her social community. The hospital and its patients and staff may, in certain situations and circumstances, be experienced as a kind of social community. For a great many patients, however, the initial experience of hospitalization is defined by a sense of disconnection from one's routine and family/social network (presuming that the patient has these things in the first place). If hospitalization in relation to patients and visitors involves a sense of the loss of social support, then how might health facilities begin to reduce the stress associated with such a sense of loss? Ulrich notes that there are several strategies those facilities might utilize in order to provide a sense of comfort and sociality. In addition to providing facilities and accommodations for family members (from overnight lodging to beds in patient rooms), facilities need to structure comfortable waiting areas with "movable seating," a garden, or sitting areas that "foster patient/visitor interaction."[38] But Ulrich cautions designers to be careful to maintain a sense of privacy, because patients and visitors may not feel comfortable with this structured interaction.

One way in which hospitals fostered a sense of connection between the patient and his or her social community was through television. In articles describing early approaches to hospital installation, a primary motivation for hospital administrators to offer television to patients was a belief in the medium's therapeutic value. For instance, in an account of hospital television use at the Euclid-Glenville Hospital in a suburb of Cleveland, television was used to establish a sense of continuity between the hospital and the home, and, in turn, to reduce the institutional aspects of the hospital: "A vast majority of the people in our community view television in their homes, and we feel that there is a definite therapeutic value in giving the same entertainment and relaxation to these same people when they are in our hospital."[39] It is significant that in this case, the hospital is located in a suburb of Cleveland rather than in an urban area, and that television is being used to attract a certain class of patients. No doubt the turn to a patient-centered hospital was also motivated by the recognition that it was of economic value to the institution.

Television evoked feelings of home or an elsewhere, according to television marketers, hospital administrators, and patients themselves; it also underscored the modern aspects of hospitals. Television sets in private and semiprivate hospital rooms took their places within an array of medical gadgetry and machines, remote control devices, closed-circuit viewing, and elaborate communication systems. As a modern communication machine, television was the perfect expression of the miracles of contemporary medicine. It also represented familiarity by bringing patients not just a sense of home, but sometimes home itself through "video visits" with family and friends (see figure 6).[40] It also served as a means of connecting private and semiprivate patient rooms to centralized nursing and monitoring stations.

Hospital administrators, television manufacturers, staff, and patients were asked to regard television as more than a mere amenity or just one more piece of technological equipment to be managed by overworked nursing staff. Through a series of technological innovations and design integrations that combined patient pleasure with nurses' labor, hospital television was marketed as an unobtrusive, healing appliance. What these advertisements and the supporting materials show is an ever-increasing emphasis on *integration* and *connection* in relation to the capacity of hospital communication systems and television to monitor individual patients.

*The Modern Hospital* even devoted an entire section to a discussion of urban hospitals. By 1967 this category was increasingly being used as code to describe not just the location of the hospital at a city's center, but its patient population: poor, black, and without insurance or other means of paying. The gulf between these hospitals and their suburban satellites or branch hospitals only grew. Also, given that by the mid-1960s the open ward was a thing of the past in most cities in the United States, the increase in private and semiprivate rooms might be understood as an institutional way of coping with enforced racial integration of hospitals. Under Title VI of the Civil Rights Act, hospitals receiving any form of federal financial assistance were prohibited from discriminating based on a person's race, color, or national origin. As discussed above, the earlier Hill-Burton Act included a similar provision, but segregation in hospitals continued. Indeed, after the passage of the Civil Rights Act, *The Modern Hospital* published several articles and edi-

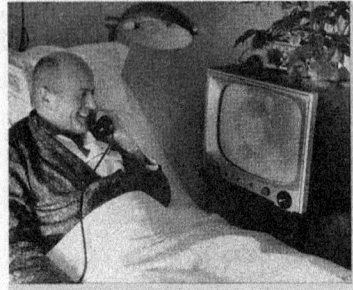

# Children Visit Patients By Television

by Lydia Bickford

*A hospitalized father is cheered . . .*

■ THE VISIT VISION installation at Morristown Memorial Hospital, which makes it possible for patients to see and talk to their under-age children via TV and telephone, is a hook-up that can be arranged in hospitals which already have a closed circuit TV antenna system.

Memorial had recently installed its master antenna, to make possible better TV reception, when a member of the ITV company suddenly conceived the idea of the child visits through TV — and offered to try out the plan at our hospital.

Ideally, the ITV company supplies the hospital with a booth complete with the necessary equipment, which costs $2,500. In our case, we did not have enough room for such a booth, but our maintenance department was fortunate in finding satisfactory space in an unused telephone booth, installed a glass partition, and set up the necessary technical equipment behind it. This equipment includes a camera to photograph the child, a monitor TV set so he can see himself as he will be seen in the patient's room — and incidentally, keep within the bounds of the TV screen—the master antenna, a telephone, and lighting that is synchronized with the coin meter, so that the lights will come on when the quarter is deposited in the meter.

Mrs. Bickford is Public Relations Director at the Morristown Memorial Hospital in Morristown, N. J.

ITV Company is the eastern division of Dage Television, Michigan City, Indiana.

In purchasing the ITV booth the equipment listed above is all-inclusive, and the booth needs merely to be plugged in the nearest outlet. Even if a hospital wishes to purchase the proper equipment and have its own engineer install it, the cost would be easily as great, and perhaps greater, than the booth purchase. We did *not* purchase the equipment, but arranged to have the ITV Company cover the entire cost and defray this cost from the collections in the coin meter. After the cost has been covered in this way, the hospital will receive one-third of the proceeds and the ITV Company the balance.

The telecasts are technically like any closed circuit system, and for the layman, is best described as an arrangement as simple as a telephone extension in a home. Here at Memorial we use Channel Six for our Visit Vision chats, since we have no commercial station on that channel that is readily picked up. Visitors have sometimes asked if all patients who are tuned in on Channel Six can see the family using the Visit Vision—and the answer is yes. In fact, many patients who do not have children to visit them have been vastly amused by the antics of someone else's children as viewed in TV!

Please turn to page 62

*. . . by a visit from his daughter.*

**FIGURE 6**

Visit Vision connects patients and visitors via closed-circuit TV.

torials discussing the effect that desegregation might have on hospital policy, procedures, and revenue.

As part of a much larger white flight to the suburbs and an overall increase in the value of privacy, this interest in the private room may have functioned as a means of maintaining separation while appearing to offer a democratization of care for all patients. In other words, everybody gets a private room rather than run the risk of having to declare one's racial preferences. As the hospital historian Rosemary Stevens points out:

> Despite a landmark court decision, *Brown v. Board of Education of Topeka* (1954), that suggested a policy of equal opportunity in American public institutions, many American hospitals continued to discriminate by race—formally in the South, informally in the North. The general availability of small rooms allowed for de facto segregation, for single rooms could be used to avoid potential complaints by patients about the mixing of races, as well as social classes. There was an obvious gap between the theory that American medicine was the best in the world (and ought to be available to everyone) and the practice of exclusion and differential treatment.[41]

In fact, the history of the installation of private patient entertainment is coterminus with not only an increase in integrative communication technologies but also an increase in what on the surface may appear to be democratization in accommodation. Discursively, racial difference in hospital accommodation was obfuscated through the increase in the availability and affordability of the private patient room.[42] At the level of both technology and architecture, integration was stressed as an important, useful, and even healthy concept. Nevertheless, hospitals were ever more segregated, in terms of race and class, through an increase in private patient rooms and for-profit hospitals.[43]

Television offered a way to make private rooms more appealing to patients, and it also provided continuity with home and/or friends and family. In her theoretical introduction to Raymond Williams's *Television*, Spigel examines two concepts that have shaped the discussion of television since the publication of Williams's text: broadcasting and flow. Spigel notes that the term *broadcasting*, as a metaphor and a specific description of the technology of mass communication media exemplified by radio and television, "was a response to the inherent paradox entailed in two contradictory yet highly connected modes of modern social life: geographic mobility (realized through technologies of transportation and communication) and privatization (realized through domestic architecture and community planning)."[44] Williams named this paradox "mobile privatization." It describes a condition in society in which members are increasingly "joined together through transportation and communications systems" rather than united in a community based on "rooted existences."[45]

While this kind of connection was unfolding, however, Spigel notes an "increased emphasis on the ideology of privacy."[46] Broadcasting in this way "served as a resolution to this contradiction" of mobile privatization "insofar as it brought a picture of the outside world into the private home. It gave people the sense of traveling to distant places and having access to information and entertainment in the public sphere, even as they received this in the confines of their own domestic world."[47] Although the extent to which viewers were confined to their homes may be debatable, the language of confinement resonates profoundly in the case of hospitalization or other forms of confinement. How might the notion of mobile privatization and the confined viewer take on added significance in the case of a reception context in which the viewer's actual mobility, his or her movements (even the simplest) might be limited or restricted? For hospitalized patients and others whose physical movements are visibly and structurally controlled by an institutional apparatus, mobile privatization could either exacerbate or work against this context. If broadcasting and cablecasting offer the ability to transport viewers to other locations and to connect them to other viewers and other communities, then this promise may be all the more compelling in a context defined by restricted movements. In some cases, the assumptions regarding television's capacities to *move* viewers may also serve as a means of naturalizing limitations placed on individual movement (where watching television, as opposed to physical exercise, becomes a way of controlling the movements of patients, for example).

### THE SPACE TO HEAL

Both in terms of advertisements for hospital television and feature articles in hospital publications, television was most often represented as a positive distraction for patients. Even physicians responded positively to the use of television for patient entertainment and education. For example, in 1964 Charles Letourneau, MD, refers to television as yet another "environmental distraction." Nevertheless, he regards television as having a positive effect on patient care because it "is a form of entertainment which is very beneficial to the patient and helps him to take his mind off his ailments and his worries." Letourneau also cites a noted reduction in nurses' labor when patients are watching television: "In hospitals where television has been installed in the patients' rooms, nurses have observed that patient calls have been considerably lessened, particularly during the time of a popular television program. Nurses can usually tell when a commercial comes on the air by the number of patient calls which come through the nurses' station."[48] Thus one register of the positive effect and pleasure of hospital patient television viewing in his or her room is a reduction in the level of nursing labor. This indicates the extent to which the television and its deliberate placement in the hospital helps to create a self-contained healing space, the patient room, where the patient can go about his or her business of privately convalescing while the nurse can do her job from a watchful distance.

As this chapter has argued, hospital deinstitutionalization was supported by material changes in architectural and interior design as well as through the incorporation of television as a therapeutic medium—an electronic window on the world.[49] Working in tandem with other design innovations such as the incorporation of natural light, interior and exterior gardens, art, wall color, and developments in noise-reduction technologies, television took its place in hospitals in the United States both as a medium of medical instruction and as a key component in patient healing and comfort. Into this microcosm of U.S. society, the new mass medium of television moved from its status as a novel, luxurious amenity to ubiquitous standard equipment for patient rooms and waiting areas. When television arrived at the hospital, however, it entered an institutional context marked by a long history of stratification along the lines of race, gender, religion, ethnicity, class, and professional hierarchies. Debates in hospital trade magazines about issues such as desegregation, urbanization, private rooms, and political legislation reveal these tensions. As we have seen, television's history in hospitals is a material one of many different policies, institutions, patients, nurses, doctors, architects, and product designers.[50]

Different constituencies, such as doctors, nurses, and patients, each have different expectations and investments in the idea of the hospital as a particular kind of institution, a particular kind of place. For doctors, nurses, and staff, it is a place of work. For patients, it is a place to undergo diagnosis or surgery, recover from serious illness, or give birth. Yet for each constituency, the experience of the hospital is mediated by layers of technologies, from communication devices to diagnostic imaging systems. Framing hospital television in ways that emphasized features important to hospital administrators as well as physicians and nurses, television manufacturers incorporated these features into advertisements. In so doing, television manufacturers drew on the different meanings and functions that television could have in health care contexts. As unwitting patient advocates, television advertisements encouraged hospital administrators to admit the new medium as a therapeutic device and as a new component of the modern hospital.

But advertisers did not have an easy task. Since its mass introduction into American homes during the late 1940s and early 1950s, it has often been assumed that television, more than any other mass medium, is a public health menace. Television has been branded as both cause and symptom of all sorts of social ills, including outbreaks of youth violence, antisocial behavior, and the lowering of the public IQ. Television viewing in excessive amounts (rarely quantified) has been deemed hazardous since the early years of the medium.[51] A 1954 study in the *Journal of Nervous and Mental Disorders* indicated that television could produce "reactive apathy" in children and adolescents. In 1963, the medical journal *Clinical Pediatrics* reported that the flickering lights of the television screen could cause seizures in healthy viewers. From these and other studies, it seemed that just being near a television set could be enough to make one sick.[52] At the same time and in other medical and social scientific publications, as we saw in this chapter, television was praised for its therapeutic effects.[53] From closed-circuit television for medical students and staff, to new methods of telediagnosis, to the therapeutics of watching soap operas, medical experts have always been of two minds regarding television's social function and physical and mental effects.[54]

As was the case with film and radio, television manufacturers played a major role in convincing medical professionals, including physicians, nurses, and hospital administrators, that television could be a new medium of instruction and therapy. Advertisements in hospital trade publications and articles in medical journals supported the ideas that television could provide the solution to challenges posed by traditional methods of medical educational instruction and also make the hospital, for patients, seem more like home and less like an unwelcoming institution. One way advertisements did this, as we will see in the following chapter, was by incorporating what I call *spatial therapeutics* into their visual representations of hospital rooms and patients. We will see that as television manufacturers sold the new medium to hospitals, they not only depicted what the ideal hospital room, complete with TV, should look like, but also painted a picture of the ideal consumer-patient.

While television became centrally important in the transformation of hospitals into more homelike spaces, patients became habituated to seeing television in medical and non-medical contexts. Television, through medical instruction, closed-circuit video visits, and broadcast programming, was a means of defining the modern hospital through new technologies while it also gave patients a sense of connection with the outside world. Through the microcosm of television, we are able to see the macrocosm of hospitals and other health care spaces as more than sites of care. Television is the screen through which we are encouraged to regard ourselves as patients, and one of the main channels through which modern health is offered to us.

*Media, like all social processes, are inherently stretched out in space in particular ways and not others.* **NICK COULDRY AND ANNA McCARTHY, "ORIENTATIONS: MAPPING MEDIASPACE"**

## Positioning the Patient
### THE SPATIAL THERAPEUTICS OF HOSPITAL TELEVISION

Dressed in a matching pink robe and nightgown, a woman smiles as she reads a magazine and reclines in bed. Color-coordinated bedside tables, chairs, a chest of drawers, and flower-patterned wallpaper surround her bed. On the chest of drawers, two bouquets of fresh flowers are reflected in the hanging mirror. In the corner of the room, on top of a bedside table, sits a small television. Barely noticeable amid the "Dusty Rose with Shell" color scheme of the furniture and wallpaper, the small wood cabinet television occupies a discrete yet close position in relation to the reclining woman. This illustration of a woman in a bed could be an image of a bedroom in a private home or a hotel. It is, however, a December 1950 advertisement from *The Modern Hospital* for the Simmons Hospital Room No. 71, a "hospital room ensemble" featuring Simmons's self-adjusting hospital bed that "helps patients help themselves."[1] The woman in the bed appears relaxed and comfortable, surrounded by traditionally feminine colors of pink and cream (see figure 7).

The only element in the room that is not color-coordinated is the television on top of the small table. The television would seem to be a key component of Hospital Room No. 71, but it is not listed among the Simmons Company metal furniture and sleep equipment. Its presence is part of the advertisement, but it is not the scene's focal point. Yet it is precisely its position in the corner of the room, in the background but still close to the patient, that makes the television stand out from the

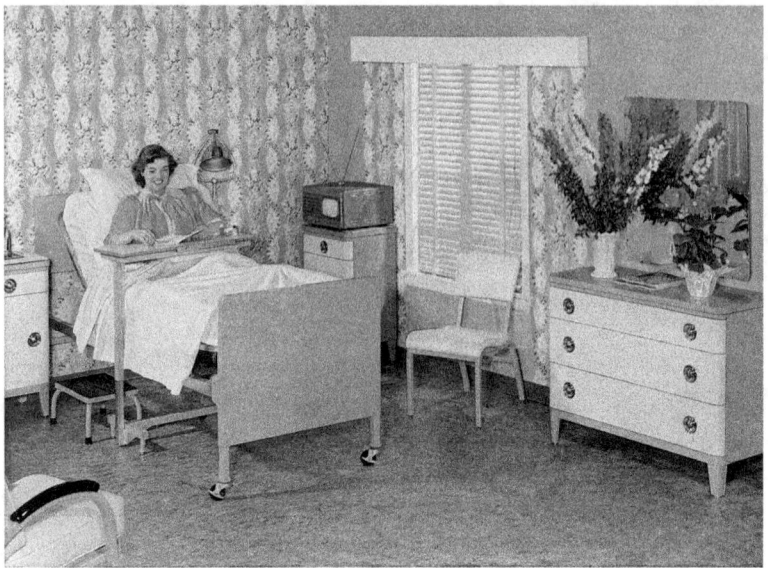

**FIGURE 7**

Television—an integral part of hospital interior design.

floral-patterned wallpaper. Although Simmons was not trying to sell television, the inclusion of the set as part of the necessary furniture in a hospital room points to its indispensable role in making the hospital feel like a recuperative, comfortable, homelike space. Based on the textual analysis of advertisements like this one, this chapter shows how the logic of what I call spatial therapeutics is embedded within these historical texts.

While the previous chapter discussed how television fit into the built environment of hospitals, here I examine the spatial configuration of hospital television and the position, physically and theoretically, of the patient in relation to the set. I consider how the representation of the patient room can be seen as a microcosm of medical care, as a space within which different therapeutic regimens are applied to the patient, and as a space that naturalizes the television as a therapeutic device. Through the television, the patient room also becomes a space of instruction in which the patient is assumed to internalize and to perform therapeutics of recovery and health in the hospital and at home. Through the familiarity of the set, the television becomes a means of connecting home and hospital and of deinstitutionalizing the hospital space.

This chapter, along with the previous two, is less concerned with what patients may have actually been watching on television while in the hospital, than it is with examining the implicit and explicit assumptions about television as a spatially therapeutic agent—one that was, first and foremost, designed to facilitate the art of healing through familiarity and entertaining distraction. The advertisements assume that television viewing in and of itself, with scant attention to specific programming, provides a therapeutic experience based on distracting the patient from his or her actual context and transporting the patient to another place, if only through imagination. As we saw in the previous chapter, television became a selling point and a way for hospitals to market their modern features to consumer-patients. Television manufacturers seized this opportunity and began using spatial therapeutics as a means of selling television to the hospital and, in turn, of selling the hospital to the consumer-patient.[2]

Beginning in the 1950s and continuing into the 1960s, early advertisements for hospital television in the United States represent the patient (usually female) lying in bed, facing the television with a remote control device in her hand. These texts function prescriptively; they offer explicit recommendations for ways not only of positioning the television within the private patient room, but also for positioning the patient within this space. They position the television as a therapeutic and laborsaving device, and the patient as the ideal consumer of this prescribed product.

Television in the hospital was welcomed for some of the same reasons that television in the home was criticized by those concerned about its potentially disruptive and negative effects on the family. While some critics worried that television would pacify viewers, including feminizing the father, these worries seemed to vanish when television was used by patients in the hospital.[3] In one context, television's pacifying and distracting effects were negative, but in the hospital context, these same effects were positive. If the patient is already sick, the advertisements and supporting articles seem to suggest, then television could work its magic as a healing and therapeutic agent simply by distracting the patient from his or her context and condition. In a space in which patients were already more or less physically passive because of illness, television is touted as an agent of mental stimulation and positive distraction, as the means through which, in its spatial relation to the patient, visions of familiar programs could transport confined patients to other places.

Hospital television advertisements during the 1950s and 1960s promoted television viewing as a type of agency through which otherwise physically limited patients might control an aspect of their environment. As Roger S. Ulrich's concept of supportive design argues, maintaining some sense of control over one's physical space is important to patient recovery and, hence, an aspect to be taken into consideration in hospital architectural and design. Television, through the remote control device and pillow speaker for privatized listening, along with the electronic patient bed that could be adjusted with the flip of a switch, offered patients ways of being active and having control in an otherwise restrictive and limiting context. Even if the only thing the patient could do was adjust the television channel, volume level, or angle of his or her bed, these movements could be important for providing a feeling of agency. In a context where others care for patients, television provides patients with a means of caring for themselves—if only by changing a channel. As a material and symbolic indication of the image of the powerful modern hospital, the presence of a modern medium such as television went hand in hand with, as we will begin to see in this chapter, ideas about the conditional empowerment of the consumer-patient.

Trade magazines such as *The Modern Hospital, Hospital Manage-*

ment, *Hospitals*, and *Hospital Progress* included advertisements for hospital television that provided parallel discourses about health and television to those found in popular consumer magazines. Considering that the same manufacturers—Sylvania, General Electric, Zenith, and RCA, for example—were making televisions for both the hospital and the home, it is interesting to see how television is defined both as proof of the modernity of hospitals as well as a familiar object for patients. Combining modernity with familiarity thus becomes a key strategy in positioning the hospital patient as a consumer for whom these qualities matter. According to television manufacturers, the level of familiarity or complexity of the device is tied to, among other things, purpose and place. Indeed, a parallel, institutional industry of television-watching equipment, such as elaborate nurse-call and television remote control devices and pillow speakers, emerged to construct and then meet the requirements of in-hospital viewers (including medical staff, medical students, patients, and visitors). In emphasizing the spatial therapeutics of the television, the ads targeted health care workers and patients-as-consumers in the deinstitutionalization of the hospital and the establishment of television as a convalescent device. The modern hospital, in this structure, with its emphasis on patient autonomy as well as compliance, facilitates the production of a consumer-patient who is literally tuned into television. Television may make the hospital seem less institutional and hospitalization less alienating. It also works to naturalize the connections between entertainment and health. This chapter explores how patients are positioned as productive subjects, even within a hospital setting that may place limitations on patient agency.

## POSITIONING TELEVISION:
### THE PATIENT ROOM AND SPATIAL THERAPEUTICS

While not private in the sense that the patient has control over when nurses, doctors, and other medical staff enter his or her room, the patient room nonetheless is spatially and clinically separated from other parts of the hospital. Indeed, the idea of privacy within the hospital is complicated, particularly in relation to assumptions about personal space and patient care. Even though the celebrated nurse and reformer Florence Nightingale made a case in the nineteenth century against individual rooms and in favor of the ward system of patient care, the idea of the private room has evolved over the twentieth century to become a common way of organizing hospital space. Now it is commonplace for patients to have private or semiprivate rooms, shared with no more than one other patient. From Nightingale's point of view, however, the ward system offered patients better care because it gave nurses more-efficient access to patients in terms of vision, response, and order.[4] Despite this perspective, near the end of the nineteenth century hospitals moved toward private rooms, for both medical and social reasons, as we saw in the previous chapter. In the case of mid-twentieth-century advertisements for hospital room furnishings, including those for television, they display a clearly preferred spatial system in which the private room is the dominant site for nonsurgical medical care. These advertisements suggest that even if patients are physically inactive or passive due to an illness or other physical condition, they can remain mentally alert and engaged through the spatial therapeutics of their private, television-equipped room.

My use of the term *spatial therapeutics*, particularly in this context, refers to how the material configuration of hospital space, and the objects within it, may be organized according to a therapeutic logic based on applied ideas about health and healing: deinstitutionalization and patient autonomy.[5] The notion of spatial therapeutics suggests that the ways a particular space—in this instance, a hospital—is structured can either encourage or obstruct positive patient outcomes, to borrow the language of researchers in wellness design.[6] Spatial therapeutics engages with and borrows several important concepts from the architecture, medical, cultural, and health geography fields that for the past twenty years have explored the idea of the therapeutic landscape. In medical geography, the term *therapeutic landscape* is understood in varying ways, but at the center of such research is the idea that physical places can have positive or negative effects on health. The scholarly literature dealing with therapeutic landscapes most often focuses on the ways that specific places are reputed to be therapeutic, such as natural springs or the restorative aspects of nature and the countryside (as opposed to the presumably unhealthy city). Research in therapeutic landscapes emphasizes that the idea of what is therapeutic or devoted to the art of healing in one culture can be very different in another, and that "what is therapeutic must be seen in the context of social and economic conditions and changes."[7] Medical and health geography about therapeutic landscapes considers not only the so-called natural environment, but also the built form of health care and other facilities.[8] Indeed, ideas about the potential benefits of natural landscapes and healing have a long history. Along those lines, more contemporary research from health and medical geographers focuses on how clinical spaces incorporate natural features, or simulated natural features, in order to both counter negative images of hospitals and, more important for this chapter, to facilitate patient comfort.[9] Examples of therapeutic aesthetics in medical spaces include the incorporation of exterior courtyard gardens, the interior use of live plants, and the provision of environmental art, such as landscape paintings or images that represent nature (from photographs of scenic vistas to images of animals).

Recent studies on the potential therapeutic aspects of landscape painting in physicians' waiting rooms, for example, suggest that this particular genre of art positions the viewer in a way that aligns the geographical gaze with that of the medical gaze. That is to say, the "visuality imbued in landscape art and the visuality of medical spaces" create an intersection in which the masterful gaze of the viewing patient over the landscape painting parallels the masterful gaze of the painter and the actual landscape.[10] These aspects of visuality, implied by the position of paintings in clinical spaces, hospital hallways, and patient rooms, are also juxtaposed with the physician's expert and masterful gaze at the patient's body. Moreover, both physicians and patients may benefit from the incorporation of such examples of spatial therapeutics into waiting, exam, and private hospital rooms because of their perceived calming effects. In some types of medical offices, such as those of dentists, this similar concern with spatial therapeutics can also account for the use of programmed background music, special personal listening devices, or televisions and artwork positioned in the patient's line of sight. It is within this frame of visuality and ideas about therapeutic aesthetics that hospital television can be understood. Although television provides a series of moving images and is not usually considered art, it nonetheless functions as a means of temporarily transforming a hospital space into something other than just a clinical site. The placement of television within this space, along with its positioning of the patient, can be considered a function of spatial therapeutics.

The concern with interior décor and a patient's sense of well-being is not new. As we saw with Ulrich's theories of supportive design in the built environment of hospitals, many parties, particularly physicians and architects, have long been interested in providing ways for patients to feel at ease in potentially daunting and unfamiliar spaces. For example, in a 1916 article titled "Interior Decorations in Hospitals," the interior designer C. Victor Twiss observes that when a patient enters a hospital, he or she leaves behind the familiar objects and surroundings that give the dweller a sense of comfort and enjoyment:

> A hospital to the average person is a repellant institution. He goes there with gloomy forebodings—with his mind dwelling altogether on his physical condition. He leaves his home . . . with all its personal touches, and is brought into a great barnlike structure without a single adornment. There is nothing there in the way of art with which to feed his hungry soul. How great must be the longing of many a poor soul to leave near him some of the things he has had to leave behind. . . . Rooms for private patients in all hospitals, and especially those for maternity cases, should be made as homelike as may be consistent with the requirements of modern therapeutics.[11]

While Twiss describes, with a certain flourish of his own, the starkness of hospitals, his plea is not necessarily for the incorporation of nature into the institution, but for the facilitation of homelike feelings and spatial therapeutics. Interestingly, while Twiss refers to "the average person" as "he," it is noteworthy that the designer underscores how attention to interior detail could be especially important for maternity patients (i.e., women). Indeed, as the advertisements for hospital television seem to also suggest, the ideal hospital television viewer-patient is a woman. Twiss suggests further that art, including sculpture and painting, be used in hospitals along with pleasant paint colors and comfortable furnishings (that can be easily cleaned).

In addition to attention to the interior space of hospitals, physicians and their receptionists began, as early as the 1920s, to wonder how they might transform their clinic waiting rooms into spaces that were welcoming and also disguised, so to speak, the passing of time. From articles in physician-directed magazines like *Medical Economics* to hospital publications like *The Modern Hospital*, it is clear that the management of interior space in relation to time has been a subject of concern for nearly a century. Television, taking up where film, radio, and other forms of patient diversion left off, presented both problems and opportunities in terms of managing time and merging space. Both time and space were understood as issues related to the efficacy of patient care and comfort, whether it was in physician waiting rooms or hospital patient rooms.[12]

Ideas about the relation between spatial management and patients are embodied in the arrangement of material objects, hospital structures, and patients. Television, as a component of this spatial environment, thus becomes another object to be used as well as a means of managing space and time. Implicit in advertisements for hospital television is an assumption that space matters and that television has a role to play in creating a therapeutic sense of medical spaces. Whether it is doctors' waiting room or patients' rooms in hospitals, television, like other features of interior design, functions as a spatial therapeutic in that it reshapes the passing of time and patients' experiences of hospitalization (at least according to the advertisements).

Television, as media scholars have pointed out, is an active instrument in the configuration and mapping of different kinds of spaces just as it is situated within and through material contexts. Television creates spatial arrangements and relations as much as it is created by the spaces it occupies. It also positions us, as viewers, in certain preferred roles as consumers and, as this chapter and the following ones will show, as particular kinds of potential consumer-patients. While television positions viewers within specific spatial contexts, however, its capacity to position us, to fix us in a particular role, identity, or place, is not without limits. In other words, while advertisements and articles in hospital and medical publications extol the virtues of television as a spatial therapeutic in a positive sense, it may also be the case that this therapeutic may have an unanticipated effect on consumer-patients. As Stuart Hall emphasizes, the encoding and decoding dynamic does not guarantee meaning or the precise understanding of the preferred message.[13] It is possible that, while framed within the therapeutic space of the hospital, television could signify to patients a feeling of immobility rather than mobility, of entrapment rather than movement. We may not always and do not always respond to television in the ways that advertisers and programmers would like us to. This idea of the double-edged aspects of spatial therapeutics will be discussed in greater detail in the next two chapters, as they address television's role in direct-to-consumer drug advertising and the medicalization of the modern home.

### POSITIONING THE PATIENT: TELEVISION AND THE SPATIAL THERAPEUTICS OF PROXIMITY

One of the most remarkable aspects of advertisements for hospital television during the decades of its installation and routinization had to do with the position of the patient in relation to the television. While advertisements for televisions in popular magazines tended to represent women as performing another activity, such as knitting or sewing, while watching television, advertisements for hospital television featured female patients not only as the ideal viewers but also, at least while in the hospital, doing nothing other than watching TV. If television viewing was at the very least a troubled activity for women in the home, as Spigel has shown, then hospital television viewing for female patients was a guilt-free indulgence and even a therapeutic pastime. According to this model of how to be a patient, television viewing enables patients to temporarily imagine themselves as something other than a hospitalized, passive object of medical attention and regulation. It facilitates a way of feeling a sense of agency that in and of itself can be therapeutic; moreover, television creates a framework for addressing the patient as a consumer of health and an active agent in caring for oneself through entertainment.

It is in the representations of space as much as in the material structure of space itself that we can understand how certain types of meanings about, for example, patients and hospitals or power and expertise are circulated and experienced. As Henri Lefebvre explains,

> We may be sure that representations of space have a practical impact, that they intervene in and modify spatial *textures* which are informed by effective knowledge and ideology. Representations of space must therefore have a substantial role and a specific influence in the production of space. Their intervention occurs by way of construction—in other words, by way of architecture, conceived of not as the building of a particular structure, palace, or monument, but rather as a project embedded in a spatial context and a texture which call for "representations" that will not vanish into the symbolic or imaginary realms.[14]

Whether we are discussing maps, architectural blueprints, or advertisements, Lefebvre's conceptualization of representation is important for thinking about how, for example, the space of the hospital room can also be transformed by our ways of being in it as well as the objects that are enfolded into the space. What are some of the implicit assumptions about the space of the hospital room, and of television within it, in hospital television advertisements? How is the patient positioned in relation to the television? How do particular television technologies, such as the remote control device, serve as a material and symbolic representation of converging space (connecting television control with patient control and the nurse-call system)? In response to Lefebvre's way of understanding the relation between representation and particular structures, I argue that hospital television advertisements represent ideal visions of spatiality and of an idealized proximity between the television, the patient, and the home. If proximity implies a relation between things, then we can see evidence of a spatial affinity between the television and the patient, an implied relation based on the therapeutic possibilities of space.

Television's precursors—film and radio—literally made room for the new medium by prompting hospitals to reconfigure spaces to accommodate film exhibition and radio listening. As we have seen, while hospitals incorporated these media into their existing structures, institutions were also revising previously held assumptions about the institutional characteristics of contemporary hospitals. Moving away from the function-over-form approach to hospital architectural style, modern hospitals began to change interior spatial organization and incorporate homelike design features. The introduction of patient-oriented media into hospitals, as I argued in previous chapters, also had the effect of deinstitutionalizing these spaces and paving the way for a less clinical approach to medical care.

Through its spatial proximity to the patient's bed, television offered a way for patients to focus their gaze on a familiar screen and to literally look away from their bodies and from common devices such as IV drips, heart rate– and blood pressure–monitoring machines, and other medical technologies. As the previous chapter explained, beginning in the late 1940s hospital television was a multipurpose medium. It was an instructional tool for medical doctors and students, depicting live surgery captured by closed-circuit cameras, or displaying pedagogical programs for nursing staff; it was also a surveillance medium for nurses to extend their monitoring gaze of individual patients; and it was a medium of entertainment and therapeutic distraction for patients. While the most we can do is speculate on how patients in hospitals may have viewed actual television programming, we can read the advertisements and journal articles for indications about the assumptions that literally placed television in private rooms.

Taking its place with other interior design and spatial features in modern hospitals, television was more than just another machine or metaphoric window on the world. For example, one of the first television advertisements in a hospital trade publication endows the televi-

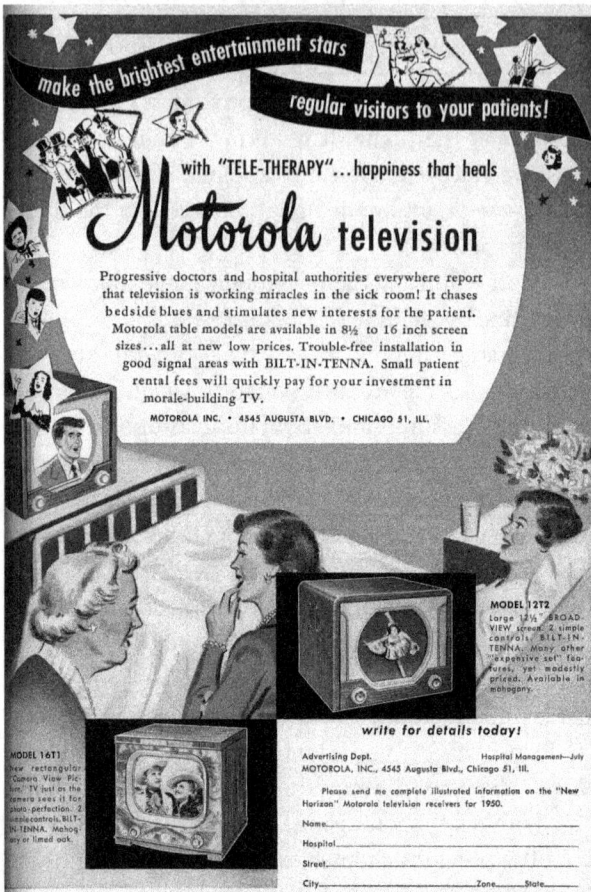

FIGURE 8

TV as tele-therapy—good for what ails you.

sion with almost supernatural healing powers. The 1950 Motorola advertisement from *Hospital Management* boasts, "'TELE-THERAPY' . . . happiness that heals," in its pitch to hospital administrators (see figure 8).[15] This television manufacturer's ad depicts a female patient lying in bed, surrounded by female visitors, television sets, and illustrated images of TV and movie stars. The movie and TV stars are literally coming out of the screen, forming an intimate constellation around the patient's bed. This advertisement promotes the placement of television and its healing properties in a number of ways, including its emphasis on connections between the patient, in her bed, and the images on the screen. Importantly, the advertisement reminds hospital administrators that television is a service that is paid for by patients. On the one hand, hospitals made it seem as if they were supplying patients with a free amenity that would provide patients with therapeutic distraction. On the other hand, television therapy, like other hospital services, had to be paid for by the patient.

Critics, popular magazine writers, childrearing experts, social psychologists, and other cultural arbiters decried the perceived negative effects of television on the family, children, and women's work in the home, yet other medical doctors, nurses, and mental health professionals saw television from a different perspective. As the previous chapter detailed, rather than enumerating the ways that television could disrupt normative familial patterns and behaviors, articles, reports and advertisements like this one emphasized how television viewing by patients might provide a means of reconnecting hospitalized individuals with their friends and families at home. The Motorola advertisement depicts that concept in a very literal way.

Given that patients were ill or physically confined, at least to some degree, to a hospital bed, and thus different from healthy people at home, television was seen not as a problematic distraction but a panacea, a therapeutic device that had the potential to work "miracles in the sick room" and chase "bedside blues," as the Motorola advertisement suggests. In this advertisement, the patient's room is not an isolated space, but one in which she is surrounded by friends and images of television characters. The room is not represented as a medical or clinical domain, but as more of a social one in which visitors come to see the patient. Television is represented as a visitor as well as a social connector to friends and family.

Interestingly, in most advertisements for hospital television, the center of the patient's room is the bed and the person in it, with all other instruments placed around it and within close proximity to the patient. Like all other instruments within the hospital space, the bed is a historical artifact that bears within its structure particular ideas about the relationship between the patient's body, the bed, and the physician.[16] Advertisements for hospital television, like this early Motorola one, draw on this centrality and add one more crucial element: the television. No other medical equipment is visible. It is as if the television and the patient's bed are the two most important pieces of equipment in the hospital room, with all other obviously clinical devices removed from the scene. Considering that advertisements for hospital television were primarily published in hospital industry trade journals, it seems strange, at first glance, that the images of patient hospital rooms would be absent of any other medical instruments or furnishings that might mark the space as, in fact, a hospital room. The ads, in this way, suggest that the main therapeutic agent is the television, and they orient the illustrated viewer—almost always female, reclining in bed—such that her attention is entirely focused on the screen. In their omission of medical apparatuses, they represent the patient room as a temporary space in the hospital and the television as a connector to the home.

This 1960 advertisement from *The Modern Hospital* for Wells Hospital Service, an electronic communications leasing company, represents a female patient watching television in a hospital room while her family "back at home" watches the same television program (see figure 9).[17] While the patient is away from home, the television is the spatial therapeutic, connecting two distinct spaces and bridging the distance with a type of televisual proximity. The ad underscores the spatial therapeutics in television's capacity for the patient and her family to watch the same program even if they are in different places. The ad says, "The family is probably watching the same TV program as your patient in the hospital. The patient's ability to follow a familiar pattern of activity produces a sense of security . . . a telepathic togetherness with the world [s]he knows." TV's therapeutic value, according to Wells Television, lies in its capacity to shape the patient's room, and the patient's experience of being in the hospital, into something different. In this advertisement, the television telepathically connects the hospital to home, mediating distance and facilitating the patient's recovery. By its mere proximity to the patient and by its promise of a therapeutics of visuality, television should be understood as a potentially transformative media space for integrating passivity and activity.

A 1963 advertisement from *The Modern Hospital* for General Electric's nineteen-inch "Designer TV" offers a vision of the hospital room as a place of therapeutic respite from domestic duties, a place of appropriate passivity and physical inactivity (see figure 10).[18] In this illustrated advertisement, presented as a humorous commentary on female patients escaping household and maternal responsibilities, a man sits at a woman's bedside as she stares past him at the television set. The caption reads, "Gee, honey, I know our set at home doesn't have 'daylight blue,' but the baby's three weeks old already." The ad suggests that the female patient, positioned in front of the television, is enjoying her experience

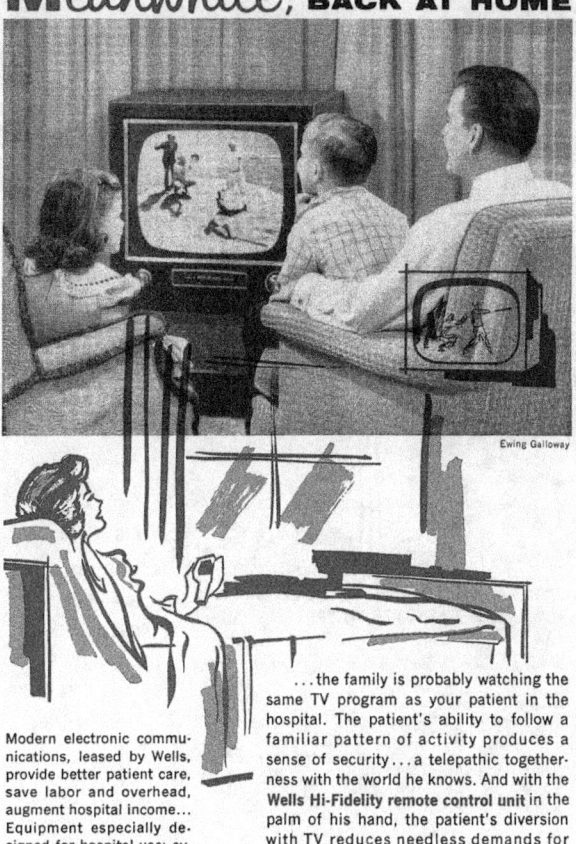

**FIGURE 9**
TV and spatial therapeutics.

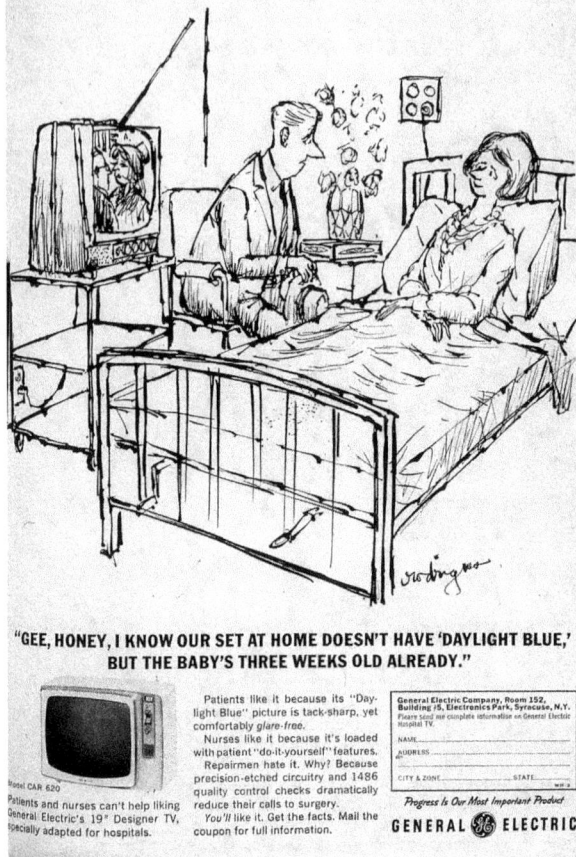

FIGURE 10
Home or hospital? TV as distraction for female patients.

as a viewer so much that she does not want to leave the hospital. Oblivious to everyone and everything—including her new baby—the female patient wants to stay in the hospital and watch TV. As an example of spatial therapeutics, it seems that television disrupts more than conventional ideas about hospitalization. It also resituates conventional ideas about women's maternal role in the home. By positioning the female patient as the ideal viewer, the ad challenges expected ideas about home *and* hospital. It also positions the female patient as a rapt consumer who will not want to leave the hospital, thanks to the daylight blue emitting from the television.

These advertisements manipulate the concepts of passivity, inactivity, and activity to suit different types of consumers-patients. In the case of the Designer TV ad, the willful passivity offered by the TV is a selling point for a homemaker eager to relinquish her domestic duties. In a 1965 advertisement from *The Modern Hospital* for Zenith's Roomate model, however, we see a female patient with a different, more active relationship to the television.[19] In this ad, the patient holds a remote control device in her hand as she looks directly at the image on the television (see figure 11). The television is positioned across the bed from the patient, enabling close proximity for better viewing, in addition to privatized listening via a pillow speaker. Zenith emphasizes that the set has been "specifically developed for hospitals" and has the capability to show closed-circuit hospital programs and receive radio broadcasts. The patient is positioned in such a way as to direct her gaze toward the television and the remote control. As her electronic roommate, Zenith not only offers consoling companionship via the television, but the remote control itself gives the patient a sense of control over part of this hospital space.

Advertisements for hospital television represent the consumer-patient in ways that do not suggest a contradiction between the presumed physical passivity of a hospital patient and the mental activity of an engaged television viewer. Rather, the appeal of hospital television entertainment is the promotion of a type of regulated activity. The consumer-patient is not necessarily immobilized by the medium, but rather controlling what she can in a space that usually represents the loss of ordinary kinds of environmental and physical control. Television viewing in a space that is as much about regulating the body as it is about facilitating calming mental activity plays an important role in facilitating feelings of consumer-patient agency through entertainment.

Television manufacturers and popular discourses also emphasized how television in hospitals could be high-tech vehicles of patient empowerment. In a 1958 article in *Today's Health*, a consumer publication of the American Medical Association, tele-visits, like the previously mentioned video visits, were promoted through an emphasis on the wonders of the push-button age.[20] Described as the first closed-circuit system devoted to the integration of "the 'self-help' concept of patient care," this closed-circuit system reduced hospital costs by reducing nursing labor and increasing a patient's sense of autonomy.[21] The patient, through a single, integrated remote-control device for the television,

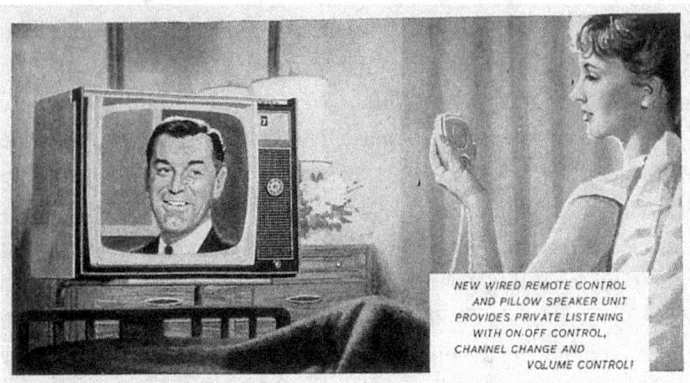

**FIGURE 11**
Hospital TV—privatized listening and patient control.

nursing station, and room amenities, could select specific television programs, control volume and tuning, regulate heat and air conditioning systems, raise or lower the bed, open or close the window or draperies, and operate a closed-circuit television system to talk with and see visitors. In this case, the closed-circuit television is also a *close*-circuit television.

These technological devices, facilitated through an integration of television entertainment with practical services such as the nurse-call button and remote control, gave consumer-patients a sense of empowerment.

Television advertisements, such as this one from *The Modern Hospital* for a 1968 Philco hospital set, make clear that nurses could also benefit from more patient autonomy and control (see figure 12).[22] Advertisers suggested that reliable televisions could reduce needless nurse visits to patient rooms for such things as adjusting color or picture clarity. While nurses were responsible for patients, they should not be responsible for televisions. Philco states that "a temperamental color TV can take up a lot of valuable nursing time. And, naturally enough, many hospital administrators have written off color TV as a headache they can do without." But with this new set, Philco has manufactured a non-temperamental television—one that "soothes away many of the aches of offering color TV" to patients. The advertisement also reveals the gendered and consumerist aspects of patient television viewing (and nursing) by offering to send a small makeup kit to the hospital employee who returned the attached coupon requesting more information about Philco's hospital television sets.

In these advertisements, hospital television also functions as a spatially therapeutic agent through its merging of patient entertainment, control, and surveillance. That is, through the development of the integrated television remote control with a patient-operated nurse-call button and voice communication system, patients could not only control their sets but also contact nurses for medical attention. A 1963 advertisement for the DuKane Corporation's "Multi-Function Pillow Speaker" represents the nurse-call/TV remote control system as a timesaving and space-integrating device, using terms such as *automatic*, *efficiency*, and *control* to convey patient autonomy (see figure 13).[23] Integrated communication systems are visually represented through a close-up image of a female hand pointing to a push-button remote control device. The manicured hand displays the size and manageability of the remote control. This advertisement foregrounds that all it takes is a single touch of the finger to summon a nurse. More specifically, the nurse-call button is situated in such a way as to make it, by proximity to the other buttons, just another channel to choose. Through the emphasis on the secure feeling of having control over both entertainment and nurse contact, the advertisement stresses that at the touch of a button a patient can receive a response. This proximity between the nurse-call button and other con-

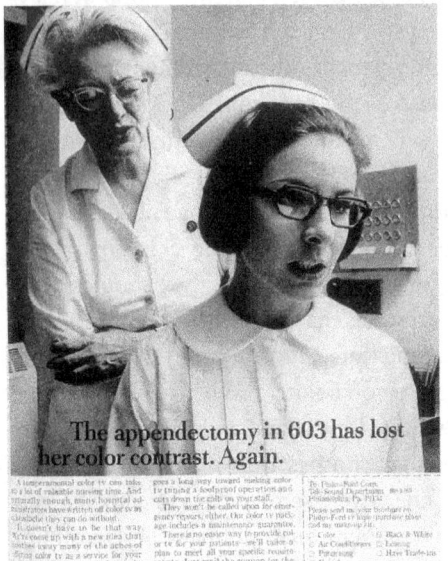

**FIGURE 12**
Nurses nurse patients, not TV, thanks to Philco.

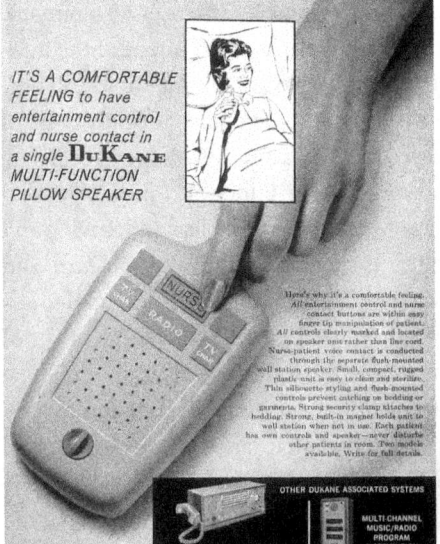

**FIGURE 13**
At the touch of a button—integrated entertainment and therapeutic functions.

trols for television and radio underscores that the nurse's response should be quick and immediate, just like changing the channel.

## HOME REMEDY FOR THE CONSUMER-PATIENT

Details of spatial arrangement can represent preferred ways of moving in and through built environments. In the case of the placement of the hospital television, we can see (1) particular understandings of television as a therapeutic device; (2) the representations of the individual patient room as a site of medical care; and (3) the conditions within which television is received as an entertaining and therapeutic distraction.[24] The hospital room is a partially private space as well as a site for the application of professional medical care—a space of labor, recovery, and death. The patient's room is, then, an in-between space and the most homelike area in the hospital. Indeed, the private patient room is the space that most closely resembles, at least in terms of furnishings and placement, a bedroom.

Through textual analysis of advertisements for hospital television from the early 1950s through the late 1960s, this chapter has shown how television, through its place in the space of the hospital as well as how it was used, became part of the deinstitutionalization of the hospital and the production of the consumer-patient. Whether it took the form of closed-circuit visits, educational programming, patient surveillance, or patient entertainment, television in the hospital was a spatial therapeutic agent in that it connected home and hospital, as well as the nurse to the patient. This chapter goes a step further to examine the ways that advertisements for hospital television offer an implied logic of spatial therapeutics not only in the arrangement of the television within the space of the patient's room, but also in the very positioning of the patient.

As a hybrid construction, the subject position of the consumer-patient embodies the processes I have described through the concept of spatial therapeutics. The patient is simultaneously positioned as a compliant subject while also offered a regulated possibility of agency and control over some features of the hospital space. Further, I maintain that by positioning the television as an indispensable piece of technology for recovery and health in the hospital, these advertisements contributed to its normalization as a dispenser of medical information in the home. As domestic spaces increasingly become privileged sites for medical care (sometimes out of necessity), as well as for the circulation of medical information and marketing, television can be understood as a spatially therapeutic agent there as well.

Just as the concepts of instantaneous response and access were and continue to be meaningful in hospitals, they also function similarly in relation to the consumer-patients' access to medical information and spatial therapeutics inside the home. As the next chapter demonstrates by the example of pharmaceutical advertisements that position the television viewer as a likely consumer-patient, home becomes both a potential extension of the hospital and a medicalized environment. Moreover, even if consumers resist or otherwise do not identify with the subjectivities created by something as blatantly medicalizing as pharmaceutical advertisements on television, domestic spaces are increasingly becoming centers of all kinds of medical care, from a rise in home-based health care to the availability of medical information on the Internet. In other words, we, as consumers and potential patients, no longer have to go to a physician or hospital for certain kinds of expert medical advice. While there are limitations to the kind of practical care and information consumers can receive within the home, it is nonetheless possible to view the contemporary home as a medical center, either out of economic necessity or enabled by economic privilege, depending on an individual's financial situation.

Advertisements based on the spatial therapeutics of hospital television offered efficiency, control, and instantaneous results to patients in ways that are remarkably similar to the contemporary promotions of prescription drug advertising. As an extension of the remote control that changed the channel or brought the nurse to the patient, direct-to-consumer drug ads promise instant fixes to complex medical problems, as consumer-patients are offered the possibility of relief at the press of a button. The ways that patients are positioned in these television advertisements from the 1950s and 1960s serve as precursors to the positioning of consumer-patients in contemporary pharmaceutical commercials. As the following two chapters will show, discourses of access, agency, and self-healing are again used to address consumers as empowered patients.

*Gone is the time when doctors held complete power and prescription medicines were treated as a sacred and separate world. These ads mark the full dawning of an age when our very health is sold to us like soap.*
LISA BELKIN, "PRIME TIME PUSHERS"

## Television in and out of the Hospital
### BROADCASTING DIRECTLY TO THE CONSUMER-PATIENT

In the *I Love Lucy* episode "Lucy Does a TV Commercial," originally broadcast on May 5, 1952, Lucy finally gets her television break as a pitch-gal for the descriptively titled quack medicine "Vitameatavegamin." During rehearsal for the commercial, Lucy is asked to repeatedly slurp tablespoons of the elixir and describe the qualities of Vitameatavegamin. Directly addressing the camera, Lucy asks the audience at home, "Are you tired, run-down, listless? Do you poop-out at parties? Are you unpopular? The answer to all your problems is in this little bottle." Encouraging the audience to "spoon" their "way to health," Lucy gets tipsy from imbibing too much of the over-the-counter medicine. Of course, the humor of this episode lies in unspoken attributes of Vitameatavegamin—namely, that the elixir also has a significant amount of alcohol, which accounts for Lucy's erratic performance. It also foregrounds the extent to which patent medicines such as the fake Vitameatavegamin or the real Hadacol or Lydia E. Pinkham's Vegetable Compound were presented directly to consumers as cures for all kinds of ills, from shyness to fatigue.[1] Lucy's encounter with Vitameatavegamin is a parody of the ways that health tonics and remedies are promoted through television. As Lucy directly addresses the camera, she slurs a variety of complaints from which her viewers might be suffering. Even more than fifty years before prescription drugs were to be advertised to consumers, the episode shows a keen awareness of the marketing of health, even if the cure might not be something a reputable physician would prescribe.

As an integral part of television programming and scattered among the pages of mass-market magazines, advertisements for prescription drugs routinely address readers and viewers not only as ideal consumers of the commodity but also as ideal patients. During any portion of daytime and primetime television, commercials for a range of prescription drugs can be found. Circulating in an intertextual relationship with other television texts, prescription drug ads offer solutions to the litany of problems posed by programs and other commercials. Not only are viewers recognized as commodities, they are recognized and organized as certain kinds of commodity audiences. Television drug ads address viewers not only as potential *consumers*, but also as potential *patients*, as specific kinds of health consumers. This chapter provides a historical and industrial frame for the rise of one of the leading modes of consumer health medicalization: the shift from a physician-oriented medical marketing to a mode that directly addresses us as likely consumer-patients. As previous chapters have shown, television was and continues to be used as a means of deinstitutionalizing hospitals and other medical facilities. At the same time, I show how television has had the effect of transforming the home into a medical information center. One of the most obvious aspects of this transformation, or repositioning, of the home as medical center and the patient as consumer is the rise of direct-to-consumer (DTC) prescription drug television commercials.

As viewers, we are bombarded with print ads and television commercials across a wide range of networks that encourage us to regard ourselves from a medical point of view. Through the now-ubiquitous presence of television prescription drug ads, we, as consumers, are invited to regard ourselves as consumer-patients in need of *care*—the care that only a specific brand-name prescription drug can provide. Any hour of the day, in any magazine or newspaper, we are told that if we simply talk to our doctors (those of us who have one) about a particular brand-name drug, we can be cured of a variety of conditions, diseases, and problems, from anxiety to diabetes. Commercials for various prescription drugs are so ubiquitous that it seems viewers are living within the worlds created by Zoloft, Viagra, and Celebrex—and indeed many viewers are. In this sense, television takes on, at least potentially, the role of the family physician, addressing us directly with concern about our health, in much the same way that television in the hospital, according to the advertisements analyzed in the previous chapters, could take on the role of the hospital nurse. The ubiquity of medical messages from television and attendant advertising texts, such as those for brand-name drugs, further habituates us to medicalizing discourses and constructs us as consumer-patients. These processes and their consequences are, in themselves, neither good nor bad. What medicalization and therapeutic discourses *do* facilitate is a relentless cycle of self-monitoring in the service of, at least partially, a healthy citizen subject. Medicalization can surely benefit the medical marketplace, but it would be wrong to assume that consumer-patients and the state do not also benefit from this process.

Medicalization works not only through the presence of television in hospitals and medical offices but also through television and other media that we have in our homes, that we see on the subway, that we read about in magazine advertisements, and that we hear about through celebrity testimonials. Medicalization through television and brand-name drug signs in hospitals and doctors' offices naturalizes and legitimizes health marketing in each space. Medicalization also has the effect of, oddly enough, de-medicalizing the physician and transforming him or her into a mere go-between for consumer-patients and drugmakers. This is not to say that the physician loses credibility or expert authority, but that medicalization in the form of television commercials both acknowledges and diminishes the physician's role in treatment. The doctor merely prescribes; he or she does not treat illness. The medication assumes this role.

Television ads for prescription drugs engage with and extend this commercial health discourse by offering a vision of consumer agency that depends on the desirability and privilege of being a *patient*.[2] Given that it is now a *privilege* and a marker of class status to even be considered a *patient*, however, the role of direct-to-consumer prescription drug commercials begins to make more sense (and cents).[3] In other words, the ideal patient is, in fact, a consumer—the one with the economic means to *pay* for their health care and the costly prescription brand-name drugs on which it depends.[4] Advertising works by convincing us that our sense of well-being depends on the purchase and consumption of a given commodity. Television viewers are encouraged to ingest a variety of commodities, from pizza to beer to over-the-counter medications, but prescription drugs can be legally obtained only through a physician. Yet the processes of medicalization and the production of consumer-patients happen not only through television, but also in other contexts where we encounter the commercialized features of contemporary health care. Further, from physicians' perspectives, there are positive and negative aspects of this relatively new mode of prescription drug promotion; but from the perspective of consumer-patients, these advertisements can be understood as new additions to a familiar media landscape.[5] Television's meanings, moreover, are not determined. If consumer-patients see television commercials for prescription drugs or watch medical dramas or other health-related programming on hospital television, they may engage with those representations in different ways than they would if they were watching at home. The idea of spatial therapeutics, described in the previous chapter, recognizes that for television to function as a therapeutic agent, the context of reception matters, as do the ways that the consumer-patient is physically positioned in relation to the television. *Therapeutic*, as I use the term, implies both a productive and potentially positive or healing effect of television while it also, as the root of the word therapeutic indicates, entails being subject to a particular mode of healing or subject positioning. Consumer-patients may, at times and in certain contexts, resist this positioning as a patient or as a consumer, but this does not mean that the preferred mode of address changes. Rather, it means that television as a spatially therapeutic medium has different applications and consequences, depending on the context for its reception and who is watching.

Prescription drug advertisements must work doubly hard to encourage more than the actual consumption of a drug. The advertisements must motivate viewers to engage in an activity that is not usually anticipated: to go to the doctor. Moreover, for the drug commercials to work, they must also provide the symbolic means through which viewers may feel comfortable imagining themselves, first and foremost, as *patients*.[6] But this aspect of medicalization did not occur suddenly; it was an economically logical extension of a system of marketing, primarily to physicians, that was applied to television in 1997. Television multiplies the effects of this form of medicalization, yet the mechanism for this practice was established nearly one hundred years ago with advertising in medical trade journals specifically addressed to physicians, much in the same way television was advertised directly to doctors and hospital administrators. Against this historical frame, contemporary direct-to-consumer prescription drug advertising may be understood as a significant event in the possible redistribution of medical knowledge and expertise.

## BEFORE TV: THE HISTORICAL AND ECONOMIC CONTEXT FOR DTC PRESCRIPTION DRUG ADVERTISING

While consumer-based advertising from pharmaceutical companies began in the 1980s, the bulk of promotion for drugs was devoted to physician marketing. Personal selling or detailing, as it has come to be called, became the major mode of promoting drug products to physicians. In order to have the privilege of advertising and promoting its products to physicians—the gatekeepers between pharmaceutical manufacturers and patients—drugmakers had to follow the directives of the powerful American Medical Association and withdraw advertising from the public.[7] Drug manufacturers traded direct access to lay consumers for direct access to a potentially more lucrative market. Today drug manufacturers have both markets: physicians *and* consumers.

Direct-to-consumer advertising has been defined as "the promotion of the availability and/or characteristics of a prescription drug product to the general public through mass media such as television, radio, newspapers, magazines, and mailings."[8] Direct-to-consumer drug advertising usually has been divided into two broad categories: product-specific and informational advertisements.[9] But the apparently new form of direct-to-consumer advertising owes its current success to the patent-medicine men and proprietary (i.e., available without a physician's prescription) drug manufacturers and sellers of the late nineteenth and early twentieth century, and to physician-directed pharmaceutical advertising.[10] Contemporary direct-to-consumer drug advertising actually engages both of these kinds of appeals: the P. T. Barnum–esque selling techniques of traveling medicine showmen, and the more tempered, rationality- and information-based rhetorical strategies of pharmaceutical drug manufacturers.[11]

### COMMERCIALISM FOR THE PUBLIC GOOD

To rise above the din of crass commercialism has also been a goal of the medical profession—and, more specifically, of physicians. As the initial audience of pharmaceutical industry address in the consumption chain, physicians have constituted one of the most powerful markets for the promotion and circulation of prescription drugs. Though not the direct consumer, the physician is still the necessary facilitator between the drug manufacturer and the patient. The economics of this relationship between physicians and drug manufacturers has a long history, but more recently these marketing practices have been the subject of documentary television programs, films such as Michael Moore's *Sicko* (2007), and newspaper and magazine articles in the lay as well as professional press. For example, a 2007 issue of the *New York Times Magazine* included an autobiographical story titled "Dr. Drug Rep," in which Dr. Daniel Carlat described how Wyeth Pharmaceuticals recruited him to conduct "lunch and learn" sessions for psychiatrists and to promote the antidepressant Effexor.[12] The AMA has revised its protocols and set standards for what is acceptable behavior on the part of doctors and detailers (this does not, however, prevent lavish marketing practices).[13]

With the expansion of the direct-to-consumer prescription drug industry, recent news stories have begun to address the means by which pharmaceuticals are promoted to physicians. Yet, without the participation of the physician, the consumer-patient cannot obtain the advertised drug. The physician's expert authority can be contested only to a degree. As many times as we are told about a particular drug, we cannot just get it on our own, at least not through conventional, legal means. The professional status of physicians has worked against the acknowledgment of this group as a *market*.[14]

### THE MEDICAL MARKETPLACE: INFORMATION OR MANIPULATION?

What is it about prescription drug ads that facilitate a reading of them as *informative* rather than *manipulative*? Isn't advertising in general always a combination of these two components? The question seems more poignant, however, because of the specificity of the product. Consumers are now, perhaps more than ever, armed with knowledge of the manipulative and deceptive practices of advertising. For example, what enables consumers to, on the one hand, sue tobacco manufacturers for outright lying and, on the other hand, to embrace prescription drug ads as informative, or even serving an advocacy function? The success of a given drug depends on many factors, including the individual patient. Yet advertisements do manipulate the truth claims of products in order to appear as if the pharmaceutical manufacturers are public advocates who offer solutions to a variety of physical and mental problems. I maintain that *because* they are prescription drugs and not toilet bowl cleansers, and due to the construction of the consumer as a medical expert, these advertisements are understood as doing double duty. The advertisements do also offer what can be very appealing solutions to serious problems, or problems that are perceived to be serious, and thus offer consumer-patients hope that is anchored in one part of the ideology of medicalization: the belief that medical science *can* deliver cures. Indeed, prescription drug commercials address us as if we are sick, might be sick, or could someday become sick.

Against the historical precedent of physician-directed drug advertising, contemporary direct-to-consumer drug advertising may be seen as a significant event in the redistribution of medical knowledge and expertise. That is the generous reading. For an indication of just how lucrative the consumer market is for pharmaceutical companies, in 1989 "the drug industry collectively spent only twelve million dollars on DTC advertising, compared to $2.38 billion in 2001, an increase of almost 200-fold in only twelve years. Over 70 percent of the promotional dollars spent by pharmaceutical companies in 2001 was spent on TV advertisements.... A total of 105 prescription drugs were advertised directly to consumers in 2001."[15] In the ungenerous reading, one might ask, of the 105 prescription drugs advertised to consumers in 2001, how many consumer-patients were successful at obtaining a prescription and benefiting from the product? In other words, do we have access to the medical solutions offered on television? Do we have the means of incorporating them into our lives, or are we restricted to watching and waiting for the over-the-counter version of a cholesterol-lowering medication? Figures that are more recent indicate that in 2008, drug manufacturers decreased consumer-advertising spending by 8 percent, to "$4.4 billion, the first cutback since at least the late 1990s," with "print advertising for pharmaceuticals declining by 18 percent, while television advertising declined by 4 percent." Reasons for the reduction in advertising spending can be attributed to "fewer new drugs and heightened congressional scrutiny of drug marketing practices."[16] As IMS Health has noted, however, the cutback in pharmaceutical advertising to consumers has had little effect on sales. In fact, as advertising spending decreased, sales of prescription drugs in the United States increased by "1.3 percent in 2008 to $291 billion."[17]

Further, the images of the consumer-patient in contemporary drug advertising attempt to erase the boundaries that have tended to distinguish the patient from everybody else. According to Sander Gilman, it is the representation of the patient as a diseased other that "provides us with rigid structures for our definition of the boundaries of disease."[18] The images of the consumer-patient in contemporary drug advertising attempt to erase those boundaries. That is, images of the consumer-patient tend to *normalize* at least certain illnesses and conditions. Rather than reinforcing distinctions between us and them (as representations of disease have done in the past, including mass media images of people with HIV/AIDS), these ad images suggest that the other could *be us*. For example, the actors in the drug commercials appear to be healthy, with stars like Sally Field speaking for the benefits of Boniva, a treatment for osteoporosis. With few exceptions (such as in ads for depression and Alzheimer's medications, where the actors perform sadness, detachment, or memory loss), most everybody featured in the commercials appear to benefit from the drug. Some ads are structured in a before/after narrative, with the first part of the ad representing the actor before the effects of treatment. The disease or condition rarely marks the actor as unhealthy. Showing obvious symptoms rather than describing symptoms through dialogue or voice-over could create a distinction between the viewer watching at home and the actors in the commercials.

In this representational structure, each consumer is addressed as if he or she could be a patient. It is this possibility, and the fear of this possibility, that the ads acknowledge and articulate. Further, it is the case, as Gilman has argued, that the "social reality of each" disease, condition, syndrome, or illness is "constructed on the basis of specific ideological needs and structured along the categories of representation accepted within that ideology."[19] What, then, is the vision of social reality based on these ideological needs and categories of representation? How do the representations of depression drugs and their ideal consumer-patients fulfill particular ideological or social needs? For Gilman, the feared, diseased other (the disease anthropomorphized) may be "made harmless through being made comic; in some cases it looms as a threat, controlled only by being made visible."[20] Drugs for conditions that are socially troubling or stigmatized (with the exception of herpes and erectile dysfunction) are not advertised to consumers on television; although HIV/AIDS drugs are advertised regularly in a variety of mass-circulation magazines, they are not advertised on broadcast television.

Addressing consumer-patients in addition to physicians, these advertisements appear to be letting their viewers in on what was once a restricted discourse. In addition to physicians knowing about particular prescription drugs, at the very least consumer-patients can ask for them by their brand names. In this way, brand-name recognition stands in for knowledge, autonomy, and determination over one's health care or course of treatment. In which sense does brand-name recognition translate into consumer-patient empowerment? By appearing to offer consumer-patients genuine and empowering information about their own health, direct-to-consumer prescription drug ads may only succeed in constructing a common sense of medicine. These advertisements suggest that the only thing standing in the way of care is a prescription pad. Therefore, according to this commonsense reading, with all these prescription drugs on the market, the consumer-patient has only him- or herself to blame for sickness. Moreover, it tends to equate good medical care with the prescription and consumption of particular kinds of drugs (i.e., licit drugs).[21] In this way, prescription drug advertisements represent a vision of the medical marketplace where the consumer-patient is in charge of his or her health. But this sense of being in charge of one's own health needs to be qualified. Consider, for example, that we are never fully in charge of, nor can we consistently and predictably control, our own bodies, much less our own health. Some illnesses or conditions are beyond our capacity to control, and thus we turn to medical experts, of varying kinds, to assist us in our therapeutic efforts. As consumer-patients we have varying degrees of agency in relation to our bodies and access to treatments, some of which depend on our economic situation. Our agency as consumer-patients, as I indicated in the previous chapter, is not absolute, but rather facilitated and regulated by the specific context of our encounter with medical care, in or out of the hospital. While television provides a means for hospital patients to assert at least some control over their environment within the hospital room, patients are, by virtue of their status, regulated, watched, monitored, and prescribed certain therapeutic regimens in the name of good health. Just as hospital patients were allowed control over their own self-therapeutic television viewing, consumers are encouraged to regard themselves as active agents in their own health.

For instance, this was the vision of self-care and self-reliance represented in the 1993 "Harry and Louise" television advertisement. Funded by the Health Insurance Association of America, this advertisement featured a middle-aged white male and female (presumably a couple) discussing President Clinton's proposed health care reform. The ad was focused on consumer choice and the power of the individual, rather than the government, to determine his or her health care.[22] During the commercial, Louise says, "Having choices we don't like is no choice at all," and "If we let the government choose, we lose." Interestingly, Harry and Louise reappeared during the 2008 presidential campaign, but this time the commercial emphasized a personalized response to health care, as the couple discuss a friend whose husband was diagnosed with cancer but has no insurance. Louise says, in 2008, "Too many people are falling through the cracks. Whoever the next president is, health care should be at the top of his agenda. Bring everyone to the table and make it happen." As Harry and Louise sit at their kitchen table and discuss health care, the 2008 version still emphasizes the individual perspective ("Lisa's husband has cancer") but also suggests that there should be a health care safety net. The two advertisements represent different historical contexts that unite two basic aspects of the consumer-patient: that, in one representation, the individual bears some responsibility for his or her own health, but that, in another vision, health care requires more than *individual* responsibility. This 2008 advertisement was televised during both the Democratic and Republican National Conventions to emphasize that health care is not a partisan issue. It was sponsored by a coalition of stakeholders, including the American Cancer Society Action Network (ASCAN), the American Hospital Association (AHA), the Catholic Health Association of the United States (CHAUSA), Families USA, and the National Federation of Independent Business (NFIB).

The Harry and Louise commercials and ads for prescription drugs present, at best, what the health communication scholars John C. Lammers and Patricia Geist call the "quasi-consumer," the patient who is only partially in control of his or her health care. They define the patient as a quasi-consumer in two senses: "First, they are consumers in the sense of holding a position at the end of the production chain. However, their choices are institutionally limited and their consumption of a full course of treatment is constrained; choices are limited by the narrow specificity of when services are deemed appropriate under various circumstances. As consumers, patients must exercise voice in ways that their traditional sick roles might permit them."[23] Consumer choices are always limited to a degree, but in relation to the medical marketplace consumer-patients are constructed as having a specific type of *conditional agency*. Television commercials speak directly to consumers, encouraging them to begin the process of becoming consumer-patients by talking to their physicians about certain brand-name drugs. In short, consumer-patients are asked to view themselves in certain ways—to engage in a process of self-examination or self-diagnosis based on their similarity to or difference from conditions represented in the commercials.

Consumer-patients are offered a conditional agency in that the prescription drugs represented are not available for purchase in the way that other consumer commodities may be (depending on one's ability to pay for the advertised goods). Not only is cost prohibitive (as it might also be in relation to commercials for luxury cars, for example), but also consumer-patients need to have the means to negotiate a complex medical structure that begins with access to a physician. Moreover, there is no guarantee that physicians will respond to patients' desires for specific prescription drugs. While there is evidence that physicians, when confronted by a consumer-patient demanding a particular brand-name drug, do tend to capitulate to such requests, this cannot be known in advance. Thus, in this circuit of consumption, the consumer-patient's agency is limited by their ability to see a physician for a professional office visit, and their ability to pay the costs for such medical care as well as the costs of expensive prescription drugs.

From an industry economics perspective, pharmaceutical marketing and advertising has long positioned itself as distinct from the makers and sellers of mass-produced commodities. In other words, in terms of the marketing of goods, drug manufacturers have claimed the moral high ground. As opposed to mere hawkers of commodities, drug manufacturers market lifesaving compounds that are so scientifically and medically powerful that they must be regulated by federal agencies. Yet the distinction between prescription drugs and other consumer commodities has as much to do with the distinctions between medicine and commerce as it does with the differences between the commodities themselves. What the medical marketing of prescription drugs makes explicit is the fact that medicine is not an altruistic pursuit, but a *business*. What we have in prescription drug advertisements for consumer-patients is the uniting of the ideology of medicine (care for humanity, working for the larger good, selfless service to the community of humankind, etc.) and the economics of medicine.

Due to the nature of the product and its ties to medicine, science, and health, the prescription drug advertising and manufacturing industries consider themselves to be above the crass marketing tactics of ordinary merchandisers. This is evident in the ways that pharmaceutical manufacturers engage in self-promotion. For example, the giant drug manufacturer Pfizer advertises itself with the following slogan: "Life is our life's work." What is interesting is that this statement is understood as not equating business and human life (in which lives are, literally, bought and sold each day), but as making it Pfizer's business to sell life. This approach to marketing, at least from Pfizer's perspective, legitimates their business practices as a kind of corporate-social mission and further mystifies the profit-making imperative of such so-called life industries.

## PROFESSIONAL MARKETS: THE PHYSICIAN

If consumers are commodities for advertisers, then what role does the physician play in direct-to-consumer drug marketing? It is reasonable to think that, as pharmaceutical corporations sponsor scientific and medical research at major universities, the physician becomes more than an active intermediary between pharmaceutical producers and consumer-patients. Indeed, physicians themselves are becoming embodied advertisements for brand-name drugs and pharmaceutical manufacturers. As a 2008 cartoon in *The New Yorker* by Paul Noth illustrates, the physician's examination room and the physician are constructed by brand-name drugs.[24] The cartoon shows an all-too-commonplace scene in a doctor's office. It depicts the doctor's office as filled with all manner of branded items. From blood pressure gauges with the name of the erectile dysfunction drug Cialis printed on them, to a tissue dispenser brought to you by Paxil (an antidepression medication), to a physician wearing a suit emblazoned NASCAR-style with brand-name drugs, the space that the patient encounters when visiting the doctor's office functions as a series of advertisements for popular medications. Even the physician in the cartoon signifies as a brand-name advertisement as the patient waits with his hands folded in his lap.

The debates about direct-to-consumer prescription drug advertising have followed fairly predictable routes: physicians have been generally critical of what they see as an increasingly consumer-driver medical marketplace where consumer-patient desire for new and expensive brand-name drugs is negating physician expertise and authority. The complaint about the marketing of prescription drugs to non-experts is framed in relation to a more generalized sense of nostalgia for a time when physicians were self-sufficient entrepreneurs rather than employees. Embedded in this distinction is a second essential feature of the public debates surrounding consumer-based drug advertising: For physicians, drug manufacturers provide *information* (although not necessarily objective information). For consumer-patients, drug manufacturers simply *appeal* to their desires. This distinction privileges physicians as scientific, rational, and apparently immune to the allure of such base promotional tactics. At play in such discourses are a series of assumptions about the presumed positive or negative aspects of drug advertising. Moreover, these assumptions include a privileging of information over manipulation (and entertainment), official knowledge over popular knowledge, and professional interests over commercial interests.

Prescription drug advertising challenges the conventional meanings and definitions of the concept of the consumer. Professional advertising in trade journals and magazines addresses the physician as an expert reader in every sense. The physician or other health care professional is able to decipher complex texts of all kinds—from the fine print of prescription drug advertisements to the bodies of patients. The assumption about physicians as specific types of readers is that they read on the go, at work, or between patients. A physician's time can be quantified in economic terms; pharmaceutical promotion and advertising structures its address to professional audiences through assumptions about time and expertise. Thus professional drug promotion and advertising usually includes utilitarian objects that can be used daily by physicians or hospital/clinic nurses and support staff, accounting for the plethora of brand-name-drug pens, stethoscopes, calendars, telephone rests, magnets, anatomical charts and diagrams, and decorative prints and wall hangings.[25]

Moreover, pharmaceutical manufacturers accumulate prescriber profiles just as other kinds of manufacturers and market researchers compile consumer profiles.[26] These prescriber profiles are compiled through information bought from pharmacies, the federal government, and the American Medical Association, "which generates $20 million in annual income by selling biographies of every American doctor."[27] Although the prescriber profiles avoid naming patients, "they do offer drug companies a window into one half of the doctor-patient relationship." One of the issues raised by these prescriber profiles is how commercial interests may influence the drugs that physicians prescribe their patients. Mickey C. Smith, a professor of pharmaceutical marketing at the University of Mississippi, explains that "the pharmaceutical industry has the best market research system of any industry in the world. They know more about their business than people who sell coffee or toilet paper or laundry detergent because they truly have a very small group of decision makers, most of whom still are physicians."[28] Pharmaceutical sales representatives use this material to establish which kinds of marketing techniques might appeal to particular kinds of physicians.[29]

Further, Dr. Ashley Wazana, a psychiatry resident at McGill University in Montreal, conducted a study of the effects of such marketing techniques on prescribing practices. Wazana's study showed "an association between meetings with pharmaceutical representatives and 'awareness, preference and rapid prescribing of new drugs and decreased prescribing of generics.'"[30] In other words, physicians, like any other advertising audience, can be influenced. Industry trade groups such as the powerful Pharmaceutical Research and Manufacturers of America insist that they are only educating physicians and consumers, yet it is obvious that they are also selling particular approaches to treatment and ways of understanding the patient-physician relationship.

Defined as a directed market, consumers can legally obtain prescription drug products only through a doctor's prescription.[31] Therefore, focusing on the patient as the ultimate or most significant agent in this matrix ignores the role that professionals, in this case physicians, are required to play in facilitating or foreclosing access to prescribed and federally regulated drug commodities. By encouraging patients to discuss specific prescription drugs with their doctors, advertisers rely on the assumption that this conversation will result in a prescription for the medication. In the sense of raising pharmaceutical corporations' revenues, television is good medicine. For consumers and physicians, the situation is not so clearly defined. What are the implications of regarding prescription drugs as commodities?

These two modes of address offer companion historical and contemporary case studies of physician- and consumer-related drug advertising. In an April 2001 form letter mailed to health care providers (physicians), Pfizer tells the reader that it has introduced a nationwide direct-to-consumer TV and print advertising campaign designed to raise consumer awareness about such conditions as depression and anxiety. As the medical director for the Depression and Anxiety Disease Management Team at Pfizer, Dr. John A. Gillespie wrote to physicians to explain that Zoloft (sertraline HCl) was about to be advertised directly to consumers. The letter included a rationale for the campaign along with a print, shot-by-shot description of the current television commercial. Speaking on behalf of Pfizer, Gillespie refers to this campaign as a "unique consumer effort," a "new communication program" designed to "encourage more people to seek help so that you can continue to provide the care your patients need." The campaign phrase, "When you know more about what's wrong, you can help make it right," according to Gillespie, "helps to communicate the message that these are treatable medical conditions." Gillespie also indicates that, due to the mass-circulation television, magazine, and Internet campaigns, physicians need to be prepared to answer questions about Zoloft. The effect of this is a warning to physicians to expect their patients to inquire about the drug. He is basically saying, "You better talk to those drug reps when they come to see you."

Several aspects of this letter call for elaboration. First, this letter and the attached print version of the television commercial demonstrate the interlocking features of today's prescription drug marketing. Addressing both physicians and consumers as ideal but different kinds of audiences, pharmaceutical manufacturers of prescription drugs market their brand-name commodities through complementary and multiple site-specific strategies. While each promotional node, from television commercials to websites devoted to individual prescription drugs, is unique in its form, the content and address provide continuity and coordination across the individual sites. The coordination of the campaign also confers legitimacy in the construction of these sites as *informational*.

Second, the Zoloft awareness letter assumes that physicians are less likely than are nonphysician consumers to see the television commercial, and that medical experts need to be forewarned about possible patient or consumer demand for this advertised product. Physicians are assumed oblivious to television. In this construction, it is not only necessary to inform physicians about consumer culture, but it is also necessary to *teach* them about what is going on in the apparently distinct patient-consumer sphere. Thus the pharmaceutical corporations see themselves as necessary mediating agents, connecting the physician's discursive domains to those of the patient. As equal opportunity pitchmen, pharmaceutical corporations construct a complicated communication loop where the mediating agent provides both content and structure for the encounter between patient and physician. Pfizer positions itself as a necessary intermediary—a kind of communication broker—that facilitates rather than disrupts patient-physician interaction. The promotion produces two sets of alliances. The first occurs between the pharmaceutical manufacturer (and its drug representative) and the physician, in which the physician is given both expertise and the latest research (along with free gifts and perks). The second alliance develops between the pharmaceutical manufacturer and the consumer-patient, in which the company represents itself as an altruistic advocate that exists solely to ensure that we receive the treatments we need (i.e., their treatment and not their competitor's treatment).

The consumer-patient mode of understanding prescription drug advertising is usually constructed by drug manufacturers, which position themselves in an equally problematic role as new kinds of consumer-patient *advocates*. When pharmaceutical manufacturers describe the ways they see direct-to-consumer drug advertising, it is usually through the frame of consumer-patient education. Although education is never really defined, it is assumed that when manufacturers describe education they usually mean brand-name recognition. Shrouding themselves in the noble mantle of patient advocacy and enlightenment, manufacturers and advertising directors describe how physicians might even have something to learn from consumer-based drug advertising. On explicit and implicit levels, it is assumed that physicians are special, expert readers who can recognize when they are being manipulated by the trickery of advertising; they can resist being cultural dupes because of their superior knowledge and access to privileged information.[32] The drug commercials that feature actors playing physicians usually represent the doctor as the expert as he or she leads groups of medical students through a hospital. The doctor asks medical students key questions about a hypothetical patient, and then he or she proceeds to elaborate possible side effects and reasons for prescribing the advertised drug. In other commercials, doctors are completely absent, at least physically. In some drug commercials, the narrative is accompanied by a soft-spoken yet authoritative male voice-over that might suggest the kind of information a doctor might provide and the way he might explain it to a listening consumer-patient. Direct-to-consumer drug advertising engages with and draws on these commonsense assumptions; it provides a dense site through which professional expertise, medical authority, and individual agency are being marketed and sold.

### DIRECT-TO-CONSUMER DRUG ADVERTISING: POSITIONING THE CONSUMER-PATIENT

In relation to the advertisement of prescription drugs on television, commercials are found across the four major broadcast networks (Fox, CBS, NBC, and ABC) as well as the major cable networks

(CNN, ESPN, Fox News, MSNBC, Food Network, Lifetime, and others), and during both daytime and primetime.[33] Comparing prescription drug commercials during daytime with those of primetime, it is apparent that drug products seem to be matched with specific programs and audiences. In other words, viewers watching the Sunday morning news and financial commentary programs such as *Face the Nation* or *Meet the Press*, evening news programs like ABC *World News* or *60 Minutes*, or twenty-four-hour cable news such as CNN, MSNBC, or Fox News are more likely to see drug commercials that are gendered male, for such prescriptions as Viagra (erectile dysfunction), Propecia (male pattern baldness and enlarged prostate), or Prilosec (acid reflux), than commercials gendered female, for products such as Paxil (depression, anxiety), Prozac (depression, anxiety), or Sarafem (premenstrual dysphoric disorder). Ads are gender coded not only on the basis of the patient populations that the medications are designed to treat, but also in terms of the demographic characteristics of the illness, condition, or disease. Perhaps one of the most obvious examples of the matching between gender, genre, and prescription drug is the Viagra-sponsored NASCAR driver, linking masculinity and power.[34] While the related commercial for Viagra consists of actual footage of a NASCAR event, fans can also watch the Viagra car during any given race on ESPN or other networks.

Expressing reservations about its 1997 approval of direct-to-consumer prescription drug advertising, the Food and Drug Administration is reviewing the possibility of placing more restrictions on them or banning them entirely. Out of concern that this advertising category could be responsible for, among other things, raising national prescription drug costs, federal policymakers are coming under increasing amounts of pressure from consumer advocacy groups such as Public Citizen to rein in such promotional tactics. Formed in 1971 by Ralph Nader to "represent consumer interests in Congress, the executive branch and the courts," Public Citizen fights for consumers' rights to, among other things, "strong health, safety and environmental protections and for safe, effective and affordable prescription drugs and health care."[35] Because of intense lobbying efforts by the National Association of Broadcasters and the American Association of Advertising Agencies, however, it is doubtful that these drug ads will disappear from television. While "Big Pharma" is one of the nation's largest lobbying interests, this conflict over direct-to-consumer drug advertising is being cast as one involving two powerful components of the medical industry: pharmaceutical manufactures, and health maintenance organizations and insurance companies.³⁶ In this sense, the health of the nation—as a nation of consumer-patients—is intricately related to the economic health of the television industry. With consumer health as the rallying cry for both pharmaceutical manufacturers as well as health maintenance and insurance companies, what gets overlooked is how the public good is being defined solely through the frame of free-market competition.

With the costs of prescription drugs skyrocketing, it benefits the federal government to identify a reason for this phenomenon. Rather than a restructuring of the entire health delivery system, it is much easier to name mass media drug advertising (particularly the form directed to consumers) as the culprit. Ignoring the millions of dollars that pharmaceutical sales representatives spend every year in pitching products to physicians (through elaborate dinners, expenses-paid trips, coffee cups, ink pens, clocks, etc.), the U.S. Food and Drug Administration and consumer-advocacy organizations are targeting consumer-based drug advertising. But pharmaceutical manufacturers argue that they are providing consumer-patients with information that might save lives. Critics respond that frequently this information is not only inaccurate but also purposely misleading. Following this line of reasoning, the struggle becomes focused on how these advertisements provide viewers with information about their health. While this is part of the key debates regarding prescription drug advertising, little has been established about how these ads make meaning about health care and individual agency. These debates, moreover, tend to obscure the ways that the consumer-patient is invoked as a means of legitimating the status quo. Dressed in the more legitimate robes of consumer advocacy, direct-to-consumer prescription drug advertising combines *brand-name awareness* with *information* and *education*.

This discourse tends to take for granted certain things about how consumer-patients make meaning from these advertisements. That is, many of the promoters of this mode of advertising assume a sender-message-receiver transmission model of communication, which suggests that there is one message in a given advertisement that the viewer receives. Effective communication can thus be measured in terms of surveys that claim to document how many prescriptions for a given drug are the result of a consumer-patient seeing a particular commercial, visiting his or her physician, and the physician prescribing the brand-name drug. What this model is not able to account for are possible aberrant readings in which consumer-patients do not decode the message in the ways the makers intend.[37] The transmission model, moreover, does not tell us how the various meanings are produced and what the implications of these meanings might be. This kind of reading also ignores how prescription drug advertising is economically significant for the television industry, providing networks with important data about which type of desirable audience is watching TV.

Moreover, supporters of direct-to-consumer drug advertising tend to frame the discussion as a demystifying of complex scientific, medical information. Rather than manipulating consumer-patients, drug companies are, according to their own institutional rhetoric, democratizing medicine. Usually portrayed as a conversation between pharmaceutical manufacturers and physicians (or other medical professionals), consumer-patients can have access to at least a portion of this once-exclusive discourse. Because consumer-patients can ask their doctors about a given drug, however, does not erase the authority of the physician. In the first half of 2000, pharmaceutical companies spent $1.3 billion on direct-to-consumer prescription drug advertising.[38] Of that sum, the largest portion, $833 million, was spent not on physician-directed advertising, but on television commercials for specific brand-name drugs and so-called disease state advertising. Disease state advertising, also known as unbranded advertising, refers to promotional practices that emphasize consumer health rather than advertising a particular drug product. Of this $833 million figure, approximately $488 million constituted primetime television advertising costs. Print advertising costs in consumer publications (not professional magazines or journals) accounted for $460 million.[39] This apparently huge financial investment in television by large pharmaceutical manufacturers can be understood as a direct result of a 1997 change in regulatory policy adopted by the FDA.

As mentioned at the beginning of this chapter, the FDA, giving in to powerful lobbying efforts on the part of leading pharmaceutical companies and the four major television networks, altered regulations that had been on the books for thirty years and facilitated the debut of direct-to-consumer drug advertising on television. The FDA's clarification of policy allows pharmaceutical manufacturers to "name both the product and the disease, as long as viewers are given information about 'major' risks of the drug and directed to other sources of information—Web sites, magazine ads, and toll-free numbers—for more detail."[40] Given these changes, consumers are bombarded with all kinds of brand-name treatments for a wide range of diseases, conditions, and illnesses. Also, the specific requirements of the FDA's regulatory policy facilitate the movement of the consumer through an intertextual consumption circuit in which the commercial text is extended to include print and web-based media. This circuit has its advantages, because the advertising pharmaceutical company is able to extend its discursive management of the conditions of reception for the particular product. It is a consumerism based not on the viewer's ability to buy the advertised product, but on the viewer's ability to have access to a medical doctor and the financial wherewithal to purchase, through insurance or out of pocket, these costly brand-name drugs.

From 2000 to 2010, pharmaceutical promotional spending has waxed and waned. For example, in 2000, pharmaceutical companies spent $2.5 billion for all consumer-directed advertising and marketing.[41] Television accounted for the largest portion of promotional spending with 57.2 percent, and print media was at 31.5 percent. The remaining 11 percent went to radio, billboards, and other media forms. By 2009, following a two-year decline in pharmaceutical promotional spending, the industry's direct-to-consumer costs rose to $4.5 billion while "spending for television increased to nearly $3 billion."[42] The increase in promotional spending in 2009 also includes costs directly related to Internet advertising and promotion as new media sites become sources for consumer health information and commerce.

Yet, even as pharmaceutical spending on other media such as the Internet increases, the relationship between pharmaceutical corporations and the television industry is a cozy one, with data indicating a significant correlation between television commercials for prescription drugs and the rate at which physicians prescribe those same drugs. For example, the magazine *Broadcasting and Cable* reported as early as April 2002 that the National Association of Broadcasters was working with the American Association of Advertising Agencies to make sure that the pharmaceutical drug revenues kept flowing to television.[43] Despite pressure mounting from large health maintenance and insurance organizations to curtail direct-to-consumer drug ads (in light of recent information that links advertising and promotion costs to drug prices), it is in the best interests of the television industry for the commercials to continue. While physicians' attitudes toward direct-to-consumer ads can vary, a study conducted by the FDA based upon two different surveys from 1999 and 2002 shows that the influence of television commercials does shape physician-patient encounters. For example, this study shows that the influence of direct-to-consumer ads on both physician and patient behavior is strongest in relation to television. Television, more than print or the Internet, was "the most common vehicle of exposure."[44] The study surveyed 500 physicians (250 primary care doctors and 250 specialists) and determined that "73 percent of all physicians indicated that their patients in [an] encounter asked thoughtful questions" about advertised drugs."[45] Yet "a majority of all physicians felt that patients confuse the relative risks and benefits of DTC-advertised drugs and that these ads lead patients to overestimate the efficacy of these drugs."[46]

Other obvious institutional formations that have undoubtedly helped produce the consumer-as-patient and the patient-as-consumer are to be found in the concrete practices of late twentieth- and early twenty-first century corporate medicine, such as the rise of HMOs.[47] In other words, given that this is the medical-cultural-institutional context within which individuals and populations are allowed access to medical care, the marketplace language of consumer-patient choice is the overarching rubric within which health and illness are adjudicated. The language of the marketplace provides the discursive limits on how our health is understood, realized, bought, sold, and lived.[48] In that respect, the following chapter, a case study of Pfizer's marketing of Viagra through television commercials and the drug's website, demonstrates the processes of medicalization and the transformation of the home as a medical information center, all in relation to the positioning of a certain kind of consumer-patient: the middle-aged male. What is also striking about Pfizer's Viagra campaigns is the way that the commercials position the viewer such that the texts both reinforce and resist conventional assumptions regarding the medicalization of everyday life.

## Mediated Agency
### CONSUMER-PATIENTS AND PFIZER'S VIAGRA COMMERCIALS

*The Simpsons* episode "Barting Over," first broadcast on February 16, 2003, parodies two prescription drugs aimed at male problems: impotence and baldness. Homer tries to regain Bart's trust and love, so he becomes a spokesperson for "Viagragain," which promises to "grow your hair and what's down there." Additionally, in 1998, during its sixth season and four years before Pfizer launched the "little blue pill," *The Simpsons* gave Grampa the task of curing "coitus disinterestus." As Homer watches TV in bed, Marge tries, with no luck, to attract her husband's attention. Rather than leave the televisual pleasure of *The Good-Time Slim, Uncle Doobie, and Great 'Frisco Freak-Out,* Homer tiredly replies, "We'll snuggle tomorrow, sweetie, I promise." Time passes. When Homer and Marge are finally engaged in long-delayed romantic activity, Bart rushes into his parents' bedroom, exclaiming that there is a UFO outside his bedroom window. Amorous attention is interrupted once more. Finally, Marge confronts the clueless Homer and says, "We need to talk about the marital difficulties we've been having lately." In response, they purchase the radio commentator Paul Harvey's *Mr. and Mrs. Erotic American,* a self-help book on tape. Yet, when Harvey's advice fails to help, Grampa comes to Homer's aid. Assuming that the problems are with Marge, Grampa asks, "What is wrong with your wife? Unsatisfied sex life? Does she have pneumonoultramicroscopicsilicovolcanokoniosis?"[1] Although Grampa assumes that it's Marge's problem, the actual difficulty lies with Homer's apparent incapacity to meet his wife's bedroom expectations. In response to whatever ails the couple, Grampa and Homer brew a home remedy sure to cure bedroom boredom. Grampa and Homer take the tonic on the road in an old-style medicine show, stopping in towns such as "Frigid Falls," "Mount Seldom," and "Lake Flaccid."

*The Simpsons* does more than function as cultural barometer of the everyday aspects of monogamous heterosexuality and the challenges of normative American masculinity and femininity. As a parodic intertext, *The Simpsons* uses its humor to frame topics such as male aging and the waning of desire in such a way as to allow for the representation of potentially embarrassing conditions. The earlier episode from 1998, "Grampa vs. Sexual Inadequacy," references male vitality elixirs and pitchmen of an earlier era, while it also heralds the rise of legitimate sexual-potency rejuvenation through the contemporary prescription drug Viagra. In its usual combination of historical referencing and prescient framing of cultural issues, *The Simpsons* uses humor to point out the ubiquity of, in this case, medical marketing and medical discourses about gender and sexuality. In other words, even *The Simpsons*, as a situation comedy, responds to the medicalization of everyday life.

Contemporary commercials for Pfizer's Viagra likewise rely on intertextual humor to speak to middle-aged and elderly men about the newly medicalized condition of erectile dysfunction. Even the nomenclature change from impotence to the vaguely mechanistic erectile dysfunction suggests a reframing of the language of male sexual performance—from one of individual vulnerability to a problem that is purely corporeal, not related to men's emotional or psychic states. Viagra culture tends to take a *Bob the Builder* approach ("Can we fix it? Yes we can!") to erectile dysfunction. Intertextual Viagra commercials and promotional materials avoid the more critical features of parody in favor of an ironic insider humor and an embrace of quotidian references, all in order to sell the drug to potential consumers. Varying from depictions of nostalgic visions of lost youth to sly humor, Viagra commercials and attendant cultural references are rich texts for exploring how Pfizer constructs an active, male consumer-patient. Indeed, as Viagra has become a blockbuster drug over the past decade or so, popular culture has also generated a sizable and ever-growing collection of jokes, cartoons, parodies, spoofs, songs, and other material culture—including T-shirts, trucker caps, and Mardi Gras souvenirs in the form of Viagra beads, which can

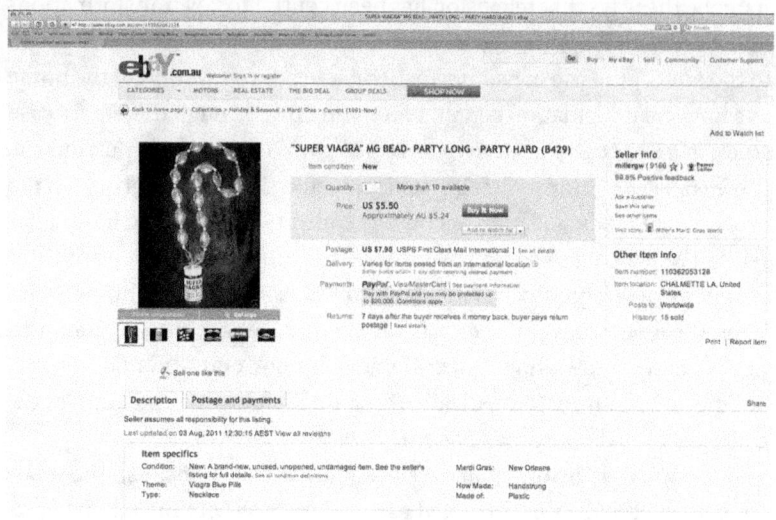

**FIGURE 14**
Throw me something, mister! Viagra and popular culture.

be purchased at various shops in the New Orleans French Quarter or on eBay (see figure 14).

This chapter examines two Viagra television commercials, Viagra's website, and other popular cultural texts to show the ways that Pfizer constructs a matrix of consumer affect in which men of a certain age are encouraged to think about their penises as more than objects of sexual pleasure. What began as an investigation into the history of the uses of television, film, and radio in hospitals now concludes with an analysis of how television, in its domestic context, offers possibilities for the self-management and self-diagnosis of citizens as patients. As a doc in a box, television consistently offers consumers visions of the wonders and worries of health and illness as well as encouraging us to continuously self-examine for signs of disease. While this self-examination may have positive aspects, it can also facilitate a psychic state in which we, as medicalized consumer-patients, conform willingly to new and ever more regulating forms of daily life. Thus the following analysis not only traces the medicalization of the domestic space, through television and the Internet as medical information clearinghouses, but also examines the medicalization of the consumer.

This chapter condenses the larger themes explored in my book—

namely, the ways that television has been central to key transformations in health care, from the redesign of hospitals as more homelike spaces, to the concept of the consumer-patient, and the renovation of the home as a medical information center. I focus on how, through the Viagra case study, *patients* become *active consumer-patients*. The common links in these transformations are television and advertising, through which the processes of medicalization encourage consumer-patients to internalize self-surveillance and self-transformation. Through an analysis of three examples of Viagra's campaign (the folksy, sporty, down-home "Viva Viagra," the NASCAR commercials, and the accompanying websites), this final chapter shows how Pfizer deploys humor and a populist, baby-boomer masculinity to medicalize erectile dysfunction and address the company's ideal consumer-patient.

Through television commercials and linked websites, the male consumer-patient is constructed as a willing, non-victimized, *medicalized* subject who is nonetheless individually responsible—in accordance with the central neoliberal tenet of self-reliance—for his own health care. The analyses of Viagra's Viva Viagra and NASCAR campaigns are useful case studies of the construction of the male consumer-patient in relation to the phenomenon of direct-to-consumer prescription drug advertising. Viagra's Viva Viagra campaign ran on television, in magazines and newspapers, and on the Internet from 2007 to 2009, while the NASCAR commercials and racing sponsorship began in 2000 (and continues to the present day). While the Viva Viagra campaign ended in 2009, the commercials, along with spots from previous Viagra campaigns, can be seen on YouTube (accompanied by many spoofs and parodies of the original commercials). It is instructive to analyze the different pharmaceutical campaigns for the ways that each positions not only the drug but the potential consumer-patient as well. Advertisements are ephemeral texts, circulating in and out of our visual awareness, but just because they are fleeting does not mean they are inconsequential or that they ever really disappear (especially now that YouTube exists). Whereas chapter 4 detailed the history of this form of health-related advertising, this final chapter specifically addresses the ways that particular contemporary medical media interpolate its citizen-subjects into *active consumer-patients.*

As an emblematic feature of the transformations in contemporary health care that this book elaborates, the construction of the active consumer-patient is a crucial link in the constellation of power through which discourses of medicalization encourage self-monitoring and self-regulating citizenship. Physical and mental health, and the attendant discourses that support this therapeutic production, become idealized subjectivities or civic duties. While hospital TV, as chapter 3 showed, positions the consumer-patient as both a compliant and active subject, medically oriented commercial texts and programming also position the viewer as an ideal subject of medical consumption. Medically oriented messages, from commercials to medical dramas, appear on television screens in many different places—in hospitals, in waiting rooms, in airports, and in home contexts—and this proliferation of contexts also shapes how we, as potential ideal viewers, make meaning of these texts. This chapter focuses on one of these spaces; I examine the production of the home as a site of medical information through television commercials and Pfizer's coordinated websites, and link this process to the ways that drug commercials position the consumer-patient as the preferred subject of address.

The medicalization of the home occurs not simply in relation to the viewing of prescription drug commercials, but is part of a larger cultural phenomenon in which domestic spaces have increasingly become therapeutic sites. Sometimes out of economic necessity and sometimes by individual choice, the home has historically been the preferred site of medical care. As we have seen, only in the twentieth century did hospitals come to be recognized as technologically sophisticated and ideal sites for therapeutic treatment and medical care. But television is but one of several forms through which the home is medicalized.[2] Pfizer's Viagra campaigns provide rich textual examples of this political, economic, and cultural phenomenon. Central to this enterprise are Pfizer's television commercials, of course, which are watched in a variety of locations, from hospital to home.

This book maps a consistent *positioning* and *repositioning* of patients within spaces of medical care throughout modern history. While not necessarily a movement from positive to negative, the historical texts tell a story of how television, and its antecedent media such as film and radio, has helped to organize our ways of understanding ourselves as consumer-patients. As I argue throughout the book, spatial therapeutics is a key part of this construction. This concept calls attention to the ways that space and media interact, each influencing the other, to produce an effect that can be understood as therapeutic for consumer-patients. Part of the work of spatial therapeutics is to naturalize the connection between media such as television and their role as providers of health information as well as entertainment. Chapter 3, for example, demonstrated how television's presence in hospitals facilitates patient agency as well as attachment to the medium. Advertisements and other supporting documents show how television was also positioned within hospitals in the United States as, first and foremost, a therapeutic medium. In the context of the hospital, television's therapeutic function is about creating patient agency and providing a familiar means of connecting hospital and home.

The logic of spatial therapeutics recognizes that television's capacity to position viewers as consumer-patients is predicated on the context of reception. The term *therapeutic* implies more than the application of a healing device, procedure, or drug to a patient. It also suggests that the patient should participate in this process for the therapy to be effective. At any point, consumer-patients may give their consent for this process or they may contest it. But if a consumer-patient sees a commercial for a prescription drug while he or she is in the hospital, the meaning of that message may be framed by the specific context of hospitalization. If a consumer-patient sees the same commercial while he or she is at home, then perhaps the experience of being hospitalized may change the meaning of the commercial. In other words, if television, within a hospital context, operates within the logic of spatial therapeutics, then this logic may also apply in a home context within which health discourses are received, understood, or resisted.

While television, from commercials to medical reality programs and dramas, may feature the same content in hospitals and at home, the extent to which these texts are therapeutic can depend as much on the space within which they are seen as on the experience of the consumer-patient. It is not as if in one space television is therapeutic and in another space it is not. The therapeutic positioning is consistent. What changes is the way that the consumer-patient engages with this positioning depending on the space. In the case of prescription drug commercials, the message about what it means to be a healthy consumer-patient is always part information and part sales pitch. This does not mean that drug commercials, such as those discussed in this chapter, are unhealthy for consumer-patients and should vanish from television. What is more relevant to attend to are the ways that, as Meika Loe observes, the line demarcating science and marketing has become not only blurry, but indistinguishable.[3] As I have shown throughout this book, the blurring of the line has been going on for a century. As part of this loss of distinction between science and marketing, television continually positions viewers as consumer-patients in need of not only prescription drugs but also other products and procedures that offer the promise of health. Yet it is this "both/and" mutual implication of science and marketing, of the doubling of the cure and the poison that is embedded in the word pharmaceutical, that makes the analysis of prescription drug commercials so significant.[4] It is important to resist totalizing readings of these for-profit medical messages; after all, they may still inform even as they interpolate us as consumer-patients. The issue is whether these are the *only* kinds of messages viewers see, and how these messages position us as consumer-patients who are, according to the texts, in charge of our own health and illness. The vision of health represented in most prescription drug commercials, however, is dependent on other discourses —namely, those that position the consumer-patient as the ideal citizen-patient who actively participates in his or her own health and, most often, can pay for it. So, to reiterate, it is not the case that television is therapeutic only in some spaces, such as the hospital, but not in others. Rather, television's role in spatial therapeutics is also contingent on us— on how we make sense of, participate in, or resist this positioning.

### SEXUALITY, PHARMACEUTICALS, AND THE NEOLIBERAL CONSUMER-PATIENT

Pfizer has used various techniques of selling the little blue pill primarily to male consumers. Foremost, Pfizer's Viagra campaigns— in contrast to Lilly's Cialis and Bayer's Levitra ads, which tend to offer a more serious or romantic frame for selling their erectile dysfunction medications—draw on intertextual humor and male sport culture to emphasize male control over their penises as well as their social relationships and individual happiness. Pfizer engages in renegotiating and reaffirming a more traditional American masculinity that can, according to the company, be achieved by taking pills.[5] It conforms to the logic of the marketplace, which endorses the fantasy that anything and everything can be solved through consumption.

Commercials for Viagra and other drugs related to sexuality—such as Valtrex (GlaxoSmithKline), a herpes medication, and Yaz (Bayer), an oral contraceptive—are proliferating and, as such, serve as evidence of a shifting cultural comfort with at least some expressions of sexuality. What does it mean, for example, that masculine sexual pleasure (here understood in heteronormative terms) is sustained through synthetic means? While we cannot, perhaps, conceive of anything such as natural sexuality or natural sexual arousal when desire itself is conditioned by conscious and unconscious motivations, pharmaceutical industries and attendant cultural discourses construct a community of consumer-patients based on emotional and medical affinity. These processes happen through a reconsolidation of normative ideas about male masculinity. Even while rendering male subjects vulnerable, impotence is read as not only unnatural but also temporary, a problem to be solved by the prescribed consumption of brand-name drugs such as Viagra. The commercials further absolve the individual male consumer-patient of responsibility for the condition by listing a variety of physical causes for erectile dysfunction, thereby mitigating feelings of masculine frailty.

The direct-to-consumer advertisements found on television and the Internet use intertextual humor, sport, and play as discursive shields against shame and ridicule. In a larger cultural and political context of neoliberal market and governmental policies and practices, direct-to-consumer drug advertisements encourage patients to regard themselves as consumers and to see themselves as potentially suffering from numerous medical conditions. The advertisements also promote a vision of health and well-being that is largely the responsibility of the individual who seeks out professional medical advice from physicians. The medical marketplace discourse provides a solution to life's physical and mental ailments, if only the consumer is sufficiently responsible and financially secure to obtain them. By appropriating the discourse of the self-health and patient empowerment movements from previous decades, pharmaceutical corporations now position themselves as *partners* for consumer-patients, as support for the production of healthy citizen-consumers.

Viagra re-centers neoliberal ideologies of self-health: if we are sick, it is our fault.[6] If we are depressed and do not seek treatment in the form of prescription medications such as selective serotonin reuptake inhibitors like Prozac or Wellbutrin, then we are irresponsible, unproductive, and inattentive. If the logics of neoliberalism reign supreme in other aspects of our lives, then why would they not apply to health and illness and the various features of the medical marketplace? As we saw in chapters 2 and 3, television encouraged consumer-patients to take their health into their own hands, whether in the form of literally holding the remote control for the television and nurse-call signal, or in imagining television as a healing connector to loved ones. Pharmaceutical drug advertising likewise encourages consumer-patients to take their health into their own hands by calling their physician and setting up an appointment, or by clicking through pharmaceutical websites for the latest information about drugs and the conditions they treat.

Viagra culture tends to reinforce an idealized, normative relationship, whether between a man and his (assumed) female romantic partner or between a man and his penis. It is not surprising that Pfizer should rely on what is known as relationship marketing to establish an affective bond, stronger than mere brand loyalty or recognition, between the ideal consumer-patient and its product, Viagra. As Pfizer represents a vision of the heterosexual relationship as once again playful, its marketing strategy also relies on establishing a solid, healthy, and pleasurable relationship between the pharmaceutical products and the consumer. Pfizer makes the problem of erectile dysfunction both *common* and *unique*. As the leading seller of erectile dysfunction medication and one of the most financially successful pharmaceutical manufacturers, Pfizer consistently shifts its ways of selling Viagra along with its ways of addressing its ideal consumer-patients. Thus Viagra, like the cultures of masculinity and sexuality within which it is both product and process, is a mutable text, changing and responding to different conceptions of manhood and virility.

As the following analysis shows, Viagra's advertising campaigns on television and the Internet rely on two dominant representational modes: humor (often through a reliance on intertextuality) and sport. By calling attention to what has been perceived as a physical aberration or diminishment of a man's natural power, these advertisements simultaneously work to restore and reject dominant versions of heteronormative masculinity. Viagra commercials (and commercials for other erectile dysfunction drugs) manipulate normative masculinity to sell to the consumer-patient. It is in the manipulation, the bending and repositioning of normative masculinity, that we can see the limits of what can be imagined as healthy male sexuality.

This chapter provides a textual and ideological analysis of two Viagra campaigns to show how Pfizer uses the demographic constructions of the "NASCAR dad" and the "rugged traditionalist" as ways of connecting to their target, baby boomer consumer-patients. This analysis continues the themes that have been elaborated in the preceding pages, while it also brings the focus of examination back home by attending to the ways that television addresses consumers as potential patients in their own domestic spaces.

## VIAGRA STUDIES AND AGING MASCULINITY

Since the introduction of Pfizer's erectile dysfunction drug Viagra in 1997, men of various ages (and their partners) have become part of what Annie Potts and Leonore Tiefer have called a "Viagra culture" that took shape after Viagra's release.[7] This phenomenon also tells other kinds of stories about the commodification of desire, the regulation of (normative) sexuality, the naturalization of the role of pharmaceutical industries as part of our everyday lives, and the consequences of this event for our ways of understanding gender and sexuality. I argue, along with Tiefer, Potts, Jay Baglia, and Meika Loe, that Viagra culture is unique in its capacity to both liberate and limit the possibilities of sexual pleasure for men and women. Not since the 1987 premiere of the antidepressant medication Prozac or the original birth control pill in 1960 has a prescription drug been so economically and culturally significant. Elizabeth Watkins observes that while "one of the most enduring assumptions about oral contraceptive credits, or blames, the pill for giving rise to the sexual revolution of the 1960s," that is not quite the case.[8] Rather, according to Watkins, "the pill ushered in a contraceptive revolution when it came onto the market in 1960, but the contraceptive revolution did not cause the sexual revolution."[9] Nonetheless, the pill and the little blue pill have come to signify, for women, autonomy and control over their bodies in terms of pregnancy, and for men, control over sexual performance. Although oral contraceptives do not fix a problem but rather negate a possibility (of pregnancy), the little blue pill and its attendant discourses do claim to be the fix for male physical limitation and failure understood in metaphoric, mechanistic ways as a malfunction of the body as machine.[10] This is not to diminish the importance of other groundbreaking medications, such as those developed for HIV/AIDS therapies, treatments for arthritis, or any other drug that makes a positive contribution to individual lives; rather, Viagra is one of only a few prescription drugs that, in its own right, can be considered a phenomenon.

As Potts and Tiefer emphasize in a special issue of the journal *Sexualities* devoted to the examination of Viagra, "The Viagra phenomenon draws attention to other contemporary stories: the aging of the baby boom generation, the impact of sexuopharmaceuticals on gender politics, the commercialization of sexualities, the shifting terrain of sexual mores, the changing representations of sexual relations in popular cultural forums."[11] Tiefer uses the provocative term *sexuopharmaceuticals* to describe the products of "a new subspecialty bankrolled by a pharmaceutical industry obsessed with Viagra's blockbuster success."[12] It is obvious that our sexual lives, along with our working, learning, childrearing, aging, exercising, and eating, are increasingly medicalized. But it is also the case that these same activities and categories of daily life are, to a degree, "demedicalized as non-professional sexual expertise explodes in popular magazines, books, on television and radio, from the podiums of inspirational speakers, and especially on Internet advice sites, weblogs, and chat pages."[13] In a similar way, early advertisements for hospital television also framed the new medium as a means of de-institutionalizing medical spaces and pleasing consumer-patients.

The main concern of "Viagra studies," according to Tiefer, Potts, and Loe, is the way this phenomenon offers both liberation of and limitation to what can be recognized as proper (male) sexual performance. The Viagra story "participates in the evolving consumerist and Internet technologies of sexual recreation and sexual self-determination for privileged men and women of the 'sex and the city' and baby boom 'you can have it all' and 'positive aging' generations."[14] From this description, it seems that Viagra's effects are ambiguous and might be understood as positive, in that they do seem to offer varying possibilities of sexual recreation and sexual self-determination. Yet Tiefer acknowledges that these pleasure forms are limited to a relatively privileged few, suggesting that the Viagra effect has the most relevance for middle-aged or old men. Although women and the topic of aging (in terms of beauty and normative body ideals) has been addressed in media, film, and cultural studies, aging as it relates to biological men remains unexamined and under-theorized. Even in journals and books specifically devoted to the analysis of male masculinity, most of the studies focus on young men, not aging or old men. To be clear, what Viagra promises is the young man's performance capability packaged in an older man's body.

As the sociologists Toni Calasanti and Neal King explain, "Studies of older men are common in the gerontological literature, but those that theorize masculinity [within this category] remain rare."[15] Calasanti and King explain the deficit in sociological studies of old men by saying that rarely, if ever, are old men studied as men. Rather, they are discussed through some other framework that effaces their status as gendered subjects. Moreover, even feminist analyses of gender and aging have "studied neither old men nor the age relations that subordinate them. Ageism, often inadvertent, permeates this research, stemming from failures to study the lives of old men, to base questions on old men's account of their lives, or to theorize age the way we have theorized relations of gender, race, and class."[16]

Calasanti and King explain the lack of studies on the lives of old men through a discussion of stigma associated with old age. As they put it, "People treat signs of old age as stigma and avoid notice of them in both personal and professional lives. For instance, we often write or say 'older' rather than 'old,' usually in our attempts to avoid negative labels. But rather than accept this stigma attached to the old and help people to pass as younger than that, we should ask what seems so wrong with that stage of life?"[17] With the exception of Chris Holmlund's *Impossible Bodies*, Paul Smith's *Clint Eastwood*, and Maurice Berger, Brian Wallis, and Simon Watson's anthology *Constructing Masculinity*, masculinity as it relates to aging men continues to be an area overlooked in cultural and media studies.[18]

Television commercials and websites for prescription drugs aimed at middle-aged and old men are increasing in number, as the baby boomer population gets older yet wants to remain sexually active and physically fit. Physical fitness industries, cosmetics, and surgical treatments for visible signs of aging are three economically booming areas—not only for physical rehabilitation specialists and personal trainers, but also for doctors such as dermatologists, who are experiencing an increase in patients seeking more than basic skin care.[19] Advertisements for sensitive or potentially embarrassing physical conditions such as incontinence or frequent urination are thus doubly burdened. Not only do these ads for products such as Flomax (by Boehringer Ingelheim) or Viagra have to confront and overcome the stigma associated with aging discussed by Calasanti and King, they also have to appeal to a potential consumer who may be experiencing such medical conditions. In their attempt to get male viewers' attention and to convince them to talk about their bodies with a doctor, certain norms about male masculinity and the idealized male body—and its expected ways of performing—are condensed and reinforced.

Viagra repackages contemporary cultural ideas about hegemonic masculinity and recirculates them as a series of discursive practices. According to Michel Foucault, discursive practices do not simply "coincide with what we ordinarily call a science or a discipline," but they do systemically organize "a number of diverse disciplines or sciences" in the service of delimiting the ways a particular subject can be understood, discussed, or even imagined. Further, Foucault emphasizes that discursive practices "are not purely and simply ways of producing discourses. They are *embodied* in technical processes, in institutions, in patterns for general behavior, in forms for transmission and diffusion, and in pedagogical forms which, at once, impose and maintain them."[20] Thus, as a means of reproducing the ways that male sexuality can be discussed and embodied (lived), Viagra commercials and other promotional materials also tend to reproduce normative power relations as they pertain to gender and sexuality. Yet it is the case that Viagra discourse makes available a certain way of recognizing the impermanence and fragility of what is usually defined as hegemonic male (hetero)sexuality. In other words, it is a subject that is both revealed and mystified at the same time. For example, while Viagra discourse seems to liberate men's bodies from erectile dysfunction, allowing them to experience the pleasures of an erection, it may also have the effect of increasing anxiety regarding a normative sexual performance imperative: namely, that the only legitimate and manly way to experience sexual pleasure is through erect, penetrative, penis-vagina, probably monogamous, sexual relations.[21] In this context, hegemonic male masculinity is that form of power and privilege that is always implied.[22]

Viagra television commercials work to support the illusion of hegemonic, uncontested male masculinity while also parting the curtain to reveal that what is taken to be natural about masculinity is just as artificial as female femininity has been understood to be. As was the case with the renaming of impotence to erectile dysfunction, this shift in nomenclature facilitated Pfizer's naming of sildenafil citrate as Viagra.[23] According to Loe, "Various journalists have suggested that 'Viagra' is a mixture of the words 'vigor' and 'Niagara'—thus constructing the little blue pill as a powerful, vital, potent, thundering entity, and thereby implying that 'the problem' is vulnerability, powerlessness, and helplessness and the solution is the opposite of these states."[24]

In other words, male masculinity has been culturally constructed as raw and natural, while female femininity is masquerade and artifice. As Judith Halberstam cogently explains, "Advertisements for Dockers pants and Jockey underwear, for example, appeal constantly to the idea that masculinity 'just is,' whereas femininity reeks of the artificial. Indeed, there are very few places in American culture where male masculinity reveals itself to be staged or performative; when it does, however, the masculine masquerade appears quite fragile."[25] Halberstam observes that dominant masculinity is so embedded as a concept and series of signifying practices in daily discourse that the only way to actually make it "legible as masculinity"—a written series of social and cultural codes—is to engage with it "when it leaves the white male middle-class body."[26]

## VIAGRA TELEVISION COMMERCIALS: SPORT AND INTERTEXTUAL HUMOR

In 2005 the baby boomer population (born between 1946 and 1964) was estimated to number seventy-five million. This was the first mass-marketed demographic, and also the "most sought-after demographic cohort for American marketers. As a group, they are the most affluent Americans, with three quarters of the nation's financial assets and an estimated $1 trillion in disposable income annually." Further, as the baby boomers age, they also represent a prime market for numerous drugs that treat a range of ailments from arthritis to erectile dysfunction. Yet, despite their economic power (although this can vary across the baby boomer demographic), "only about 10 percent of advertising is directed at the 50-plus market." But Madison Avenue is finally realizing that baby boomers, and those just a few years older and younger, are a lucrative market for everything from beer to financial planning services to Viagra. One key feature of marketing to baby boomers, and subcategories such as the NASCAR dad or the rugged traditionalist, is the use of familiar popular cultural references within the advertisements. This referencing technique can be seen in, for example, the use of David Bowie's "Rebel, Rebel" in an iPod commercial or Led Zeppelin's "Rock and Roll" in a Cadillac ad.[27]

In particular, the NASCAR dad and the rugged traditionalist subcategories of the baby boomer population could also be said to represent the social and class codings of the middle-aged, white male fans of Bruce Springsteen. For example, during a 2009 Springsteen concert, one could purchase a souvenir T-shirt that proudly declared "Viagra takin'" as an ironic signifier of sexual vitality in men's later years (figure 15). Accord-

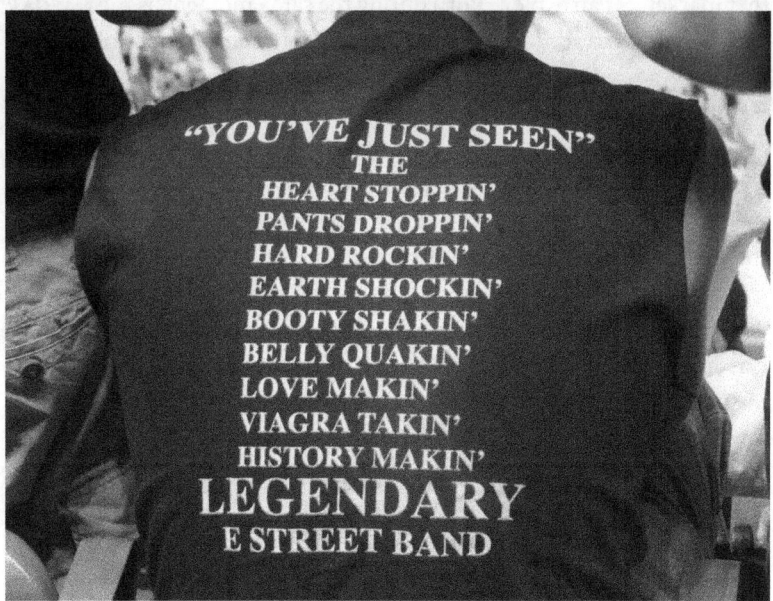

**FIGURE 15**

Rock-and-roll—rearticulating Viagra and masculinity at a Bruce Springsteen and the E Street Band concert, July 2008. Courtesy of Elizabeth Snyder.

ing to the *New York Times*, "soccer moms" and "NASCAR dads" have their origins in the 2004 presidential campaign. The NASCAR dad signifies "the white, heterosexual embodiment of the swing voter," comprising a complicated series of contradictions. This figure

wears khakis and cords and polo shirts, sleeveless T's and cutoffs and souvenir hats. He's bearded and clean shaven, short and long, fat and lean, drunk out of his mind and sober as a Stoic. He wears a mullet; no, he doesn't. He's neat as a Marine; he looks like the last man out of a mine collapse. Sometimes he throws Mardi Gras beads at your wife and yells at her to take off her blouse. Other mornings, the sun tipping the first brightness over the lip of the grandstands, throwing hard shadows, he kneels in a group with the other NASCAR dads and prays. Race day is Sunday, after all.[28]

Like the NASCAR dad, the rugged traditionalist is, first and foremost, a marketing category that stands in for a variety of lifestyle characteristics that marketers can exploit. Born during the same moment as the NASCAR dad, the rugged traditionalist is a "typical manly man. They drink domestic beer. They watch football. They work on their cars. They come home from what's usually a blue-collar job to dinner on the table. . . . Most closely aligned with NASCAR Dads . . . Rugged Traditionalists watch NASCAR on television, they go to the racetracks in person, and they listen to it on the radio."[29] While the Rolling Stones and Bruce Springsteen and the E Street Band continue to pack stadiums and Paul McCartney is almost seventy years old, Viagra's campaigns seeks this market through advertising strategies that interpolate white, working-class and middle-class men over the age of forty. The rugged traditionalists seem to be part of the same demographic that would attend Rolling Stones or Bruce Springsteen concerts and who, along with Paul McCartney and the other musicians, are aging. As the concert spectator's shirt makes clear, "Viagra-takin'" is naturalized as a practice along with other lifestyle categories.

Recent images in popular magazine advertisements, television commercials, and websites for Viagra incorporate the visual iconographies of hegemonic masculinity. Yet these same texts also offer an additional mode of address in relation to it: humor in the form of intertextual reference, as well as sport and celebrity sponsorship and endorsement. Not necessarily a counter-hegemonic vision of masculinity, nonetheless some of Viagra's commercials from the last decade offer recodings of conventional masculinity made available through intertextuality and humor.[30] Kelly Simmons, a consultant who studies sex issues in marketing for Tierney Communications, an advertising and public relations company in Philadelphia, observed, "It would be lovely to see them [Pfizer] use more humor."[31] Indeed, Pfizer seems to have followed this advice with the consistent use of humor and invocation of rugged masculinity in its advertising campaigns for Viagra. Simmons notes that many of the advertisements for erectile dysfunction are either too serious or too technical and that, to be more effective and establish a deeper, relational bond with the ideal consumer, pharmaceutical companies should use humor—specifically George Carlin, because, according to Simmons, "he'd be hysterical and he's the right age."[32] This bond that Simmons describes is precisely what Pfizer articulates through relationship marketing and intertextual referencing, or the deliberate quoting from other popular cultural texts, to articulate two visions: one supports "values like romance, courage, power, and rugged individualism," while another offers a form of masculinity based on relations among men, one capable of laughing at itself, of not taking itself quite so seriously.[33] As Loe and Baglia have pointed out in their studies of Viagra's advertising from 1998 through 2005, the overarching strategy for Pfizer was one that relied on stereotypical tropes of heterosexual romance and conventional male interests such as sports. Yet, while Baglia does address the figures of the sportsman and the stud in Viagra print advertisements and television commercials, neither he nor Loe address the ways that these ads work through intertextual referencing and humor.[34]

One of the most significant hurdles that Pfizer had to clear when developing its different campaigns was the embarrassment that frequently accompanies discussions of male erectile dysfunction. As Janice Lipsky, a key member of the Viagra marketing division at Pfizer put it, "Our job is to communicate to men so they don't feel so embarrassed. Viagra advertising is very targeted to men's habits. For medication, it's a higher-involvement marketing message. People are passionate about their condition, and education can help men overcome a barrier for treatment."[35] In contrast to those for Cialis and Levitra, ads for Viagra—with NASCAR sponsorship, the former baseball star Rafael Palmeiro as a spokesperson, and quotations from musicals such as *Singin' in the Rain* (1952) and *Viva Las Vegas* (1964)—seem willing to use humor and masculine leisure activities to re-signify erectile dysfunction. The ads that reference sports suggest that if Palmeiro and the NASCAR driver Mark Martin admit to having used Viagra for erectile dysfunction, then sports fans and other regular guys can at least talk to their doctors about it. As Baglia observes, "When it comes to marketing products, the male sports hero has no equal. What makes the Palmeiro commercial especially interesting is the way professional baseball is used to sell sexual identity to men who are at an age when they have to admit that their childhood ambition of playing baseball in the majors can now only be fantasy. And yet they still want to hit home runs."[36]

Baseball is not the only sport with a populist resonance. Pfizer, in a keen example of the drug company's courting of middle-aged men through folksy, non-high-fallutin' reference, has sponsored a NASCAR driver since 2000. Eschewing football in favor of other sports such as NASCAR and baseball, Pfizer provides health screenings called "Pfizer Tuneups for Life" at races and was an official sponsor of Major League Baseball.[37] Prior to GlaxoSmithKline's $6 million deal with the National Football League for the rights to advertise Levitra in 2003, the organization "had refused to allow pharmaceutical companies to join its list of corporate sponsors, leaving the drug makers in the same ranks as producers of hard liquor and firearm makers. The league decided to change that in February [2003] when it told its teams that they could make deals with drug companies."[38]

With the start of the NASCAR sponsorship in 2000, Pfizer began to expand its marketing campaign to include men "between the ages of 40 and 59. According to IMS Health, a health care information company, about 50 percent of patients talking to their doctors about Viagra were in that age group last year [2001] up from 42 percent in 1998."[39] Pfizer's sponsorship of Martin, forty-three years old when Viagra's brand name appeared on his Ford Taurus, was directed toward middle-aged men, with the intention of increasing sales of the drug to younger men and to rearticulating Viagra from a "techno-fix" to a "techno-boost."[40]

Viagra's sponsorship of NASCAR is an example of the use of the codes of conventional masculinity, but it also relies on the body-as-machine metaphor. When Dr. Harry Fisch, professor of clinical urology at Columbia University, used the metaphor that "the penis is the dipstick of the body's health" in a CNN interview regarding men's reluctance to seek medical treatment, he was using a similar cultural code as Pfizer uses in its sponsorship of NASCAR.[41] The Viagra commercials use these codes and metaphors as they draw on sport culture and the blue-collar, populist connotations of NASCAR to target male consumer-patients.

One of the NASCAR commercials featuring Mark Martin draws an explicit comparison between the enhanced engine of the racecar and the enhanced body of the potential Viagra consumer. Beginning with the sounds of rock-and-roll—guitars and drums—and a zooming racecar cruising around a track, a male voice-over asks, "Thinking about trying Viagra? It's now available from your doctor in a free six-pill sample pack." As the voice-over gives this information, the screen splits into six parts, emphasizing the "six-pill sample pack" and intertextual references to other kinds of six-packs, such as beer or tight abdominal muscles. The voice-over suggests that this six-pack is easy, that it's available from a doctor, and that it's free. Plus the use of the word "sample" suggests that there is no commitment to the prescription drug and that one might not even need it.

Having grown up with television and contemporary advertising, the baby boomer population represented by NASCAR dads and rugged traditionalists are familiar with conventional marketing strategies and, in the case of Viagra, are wary of suggestions of masculine vulnerability. With this skittishness in mind, Pfizer's NASCAR and Viva Viagra campaigns have addressed male consumer-patients as *active* subjects who are part of a larger masculine brotherhood based, in part, on the self-reliance discourses offered by neoliberalism. If neoliberalism is founded on the concept of the self-governing, self-reliant subject, then how does Pfizer convince male consumer-patients that they should rely on the little blue pill for optimal sexual performance? The answer is in the approaches of the campaigns themselves, which celebrate the self-governing subject while placing him in a context of other, ordinary men, "just like him." Pfizer recognized that in order to promote Viagra, the company had to establish more than a bond between the consumer-patient and the brand-name drug: they had to simulate a community of active, self-reliant users who formed a relationship with the drug manufacturer. In other words, the processes of medicalization worked themselves into the quotidian practices of their ideal subjects of address and became part of their lives. This was largely accomplished through the processes of relationship marketing that stressed, among other things, an active role for consumer-patients.

### RELATIONSHIP MARKETING AND MEDICALIZATION: LIVING WITHIN THE VIAGRA BRAND

The Viagra commercial featuring Martin and the Pfizer "Tuneup for Life" traveling health clinic provide examples of relationship marketing as a means of medicalizing consumer-patients and their everyday lives. These types of ad campaigns create a marketing environment that encourages the target demographic to *live within the brand*. This idea of "brand community" has its roots in a specific marketing methodology referred to as "relationship marketing," which relies on the creation of "a customer-experiential perspective [as] a fabric of relationships in which the customer is situated."[42] In brand communities, marketers develop strategies through which a community of consumers interacts within the context that the corporation creates. These kinds of interactions bring together not only representatives from a given corporation, but also individual consumers who are asked to share experiences while engaging with the product. In the case of Pfizer, the "Tuneup for Life" traveling health clinic might be an example of the construction of a community of consumers that naturalizes the relationship among medical professionals, marketers, Pfizer, and the brand name Viagra.

Community-building features of relationship marketing also can be found on corporate websites that encourage their users to play games designed by the corporation or submit do-it-yourself commercials as testimonials for the product. The Viagra websites are also a forum through which consumer-patients and others communicate with one another and with medical professionals about the drug. Relationship marketing and building a brand community work together to produce a seamless world where the consumer is invited to participate, and in which his or her ideas are legitimated and recognized as expertise.

Barbara Bund Jackson observes in *Winning and Keeping Industrial Customers*, "Customers are the basis of successful marketing. Industrial marketing practitioners, especially, have long known the value of being *close to their customers*. . . . Relationships between industrial vendors and individual customer accounts are frequently *close, long lasting,* and *important to both parties.* But not all customer *relationships last.*" She defines relationship marketing as "marketing oriented toward *strong, lasting* relationships with individual accounts."[43] What is striking about the above quotation is the common way of describing a *marketing* relationship between supplier and buyer (whether in a wholesale or retail context) and the common way of describing *romantic* relationships. When considering the ways that Pfizer markets Viagra through the building of brand community and relationship marketing, this is even more interesting because of the nature of the advertised product: a pill that facilitates sexual pleasure, whether for individuals or, in what seems to be the preferred marketing message, for heterosexual, monogamous, couples. This form of relationship marketing, as represented by Viagra's strategies, builds a discourse of connection and support through the sexualization of the older man that, in turn, facilitates a feeling of care that is articulated through Pfizer as a supportive corporation.

As another method of building brand community around Viagra, in July 2007 Pfizer launched its Viva Viagra thirty-second television commercial during the NBC *Nightly News*. Described by the trade publication *Medical Marketing and Media* as taking a "playful approach" to its star product, Pfizer also makes an intertextual reference to the 1964 Elvis Presley musical *Viva Las Vegas* as well as the connotations of sexual liberation and frivolity associated with the city famous for the slogan "What happens in Vegas, stays in Vegas."[44] That Pfizer uses "viva" in its new slogan is also significant as the Spanish-speaking or bilingual audiences continue to increase in size and value for marketers.[45] Pfizer's

Viva Viagra commercial begins with an interior shot of a group of men in their forties and fifties playing music (guitars, stand-up bass, piano, and drums) in a roadhouse or bar. The lighting looks natural as it streams in through the windows. The men are dressed very causally, in Hawaiian print, short-sleeved shirts and shorts or jeans. They look as if they are rehearsing for a later performance. As the first singer counts off and begins to sing the first lyrics of the theme song, "Viva Viagra," the camera shows a white man in medium close-up holding a guitar. Next, as the song continues, the camera cuts to an extreme close-up of the hands of an African American piano player. The camera pulls back to show an African American drummer, then cuts to a white guitar player, who takes over the lyrics from the first singer. The camera alternates between medium shots of the entire group and close-ups of the individual band members taking turns singing the theme song.[46]

As the male voice-over describes dosing directions and some of the possible side effects of taking Viagra, the band continues to play and some of the information from the voice-over appears superimposed over the image. The final shot is of the men getting in their vehicles and driving away in a cloud of dust, hurrying to get home (as the lyrics to the song indicate). Over the final image of the dust cloud, the brand name and slogan, "Viva Viagra"—along with the generic name (sildenafil citrate) and Viagra.com, as well as Pfizer's logo and toll-free telephone number—appear in Viagra's signature blue. With a nod to Elvis Presley's 1964 film and corresponding hit song, the commercial's theme song directly borrows the melody while substituting different lyrics—a monogamy makeover. Both "Viva Las Vegas" and "Viva Viagra" use double-entendre to suggest the sexual adventure (though not too adventurous) and pleasures to be found waiting at home.[47] The lyrics describe how the musicians have been "on the road" and are anxious to get home to see their "heart's desire," defying the stereotype of the straying musician. Interestingly, as opposed to video commercials on Viagra's official website, no women appear in this television spot, just this group of guys extolling the benefits of Viagra and domestic, sexual bliss. During the same period that the TV commercial ran, Viagra's website featured a different video commercial using the same song. During this ad, a location and time are given in order to suggest that the musicians are working late and goofing around in between recordings. "Nashville: 1:22 a.m." appears to let us know that they are working in the country music capital, home of the Grand Ole Opry and famous recording studios. While not Elvis's home in Memphis, it is nonetheless effective in making linkages between "the King" and his music—the young Elvis's vitality and pleasures of performance—and this group of musicians.

Pfizer's commercial demonstrates not only intertextuality but humor as well. Presley, an icon of sexuality, was also known to use various prescription drugs that more than likely contributed to his death at age forty-two in 1977. Although it is probably unintended, "Viva Viagra" brings together two textual references: the Presley film and contemporary car racing culture. The film *Viva Las Vegas* takes place during the Las Vegas Grand Prix, in which the driver Lucky Jackson (played by Presley) cannot afford to buy a new engine for his racecar.[48] The lyrics to "Viva Las Vegas" and "Viva Viagra" contrast to the extent that the original song is all about the pleasures to be had roaming the city of Las Vegas, gambling and chasing women.[49] If the dice "stay hot" and the gambler has a "strong heart and a nerve of steel," a fellow can have a lot of fun in Las Vegas. With "Viva Viagra," the pleasures are closer to home as the musicians sing the praises of simple, monogamous sexual bliss and contentment made possible, of course, by Viagra. The intertextual references to racecar culture also signal Pfizer's previous commercials featuring the NASCAR driver Mark Martin, who never loses his engine. As Lucky Jackson wins the Grand Prix and Rusty Martin, so too can the male consumer-patient be a winner in the bedroom. The euphemisms need little explanation. The intertextual referencing indicates that although the film shows the domestication of Lucky, the commercial points to a utopian vision of the aging male maintaining sexual practices commonly associated with younger men.

In each of the Viagra texts and intertexts, from NASCAR to Elvis, the idea of performance is essential. Whether it is Mark Martin winning a NASCAR race, Lucky Jackson finding an engine and winning the Las Vegas Grand Prix, or the musicians performing their song, male performance is the subject of each of these intertextual representations. In order to win the Las Vegas Grand Prix, Lucky needs both his engine and the seductive charm of Rusty Martin; in order for the musicians in "Viva Viagra" to perform well, they must rehearse and also take Viagra for successful sexual performance.[50] Key to their performance is the idea of the sexual male body as a machine that needs a tuneup from time to time, referring back to the NASCAR commercial and the "Tuneup for Life" events. Viagra supplies the lost engine, the enhancement needed to win the race in terms of normative sexual performance; this metaphor of finishing the race reinforces a goal-driven ideology of male sexuality. By referencing the Elvis Presley musical, moreover, Pfizer deploys humor to suggest the pleasures to be had by men taking Viagra, so much pleasure in fact that they are inspired to sing about it.[51]

As another link in the consumer-patient circuit, from 2007 to 2009 Pfizer's website was called the "Viagra® Official Site—Viva Viagra."[52] This continuation of the Viva Viagra theme is an example of more than sophisticated intertextuality and relationship marketing that moves consumers from website, to television commercial, to magazines, and back again. It also represents the melding of participatory consumer spectatorship and relationship marketing. Viva Viagra's website uses the signature "Viagra blue" and arranges health-related topics along the left side of the screen, including such clickable tabs as "About Erectile Dysfunction," "Rate Your Sexual Health," "About Viagra," "Getting a Prescription," "Taking Viagra," "Save on Viagra," and "Viva Viagra." Under this list of topics are also areas where consumers can receive further information among headings such as "Common Questions," "My Value Card," and a section specifically devoted to partners (called "For Partners").

The "Viva Viagra" link takes consumers to five possible TV spots, each of which has, in one form or another, appeared on broadcast and cable networks. Consumers can select sixty-second TV spots called "Dazzle," "Surprise," "Breakaway," "Nashville," and "Anniversary." The website is an example of participatory, relational marketing because of the ways it encourages and even rewards consumers not only for their passing interest in the drug, but also for their action in obtaining a prescription from their doctors. Consumers are directed, moreover, to rate their sexual health by taking a short, multiple-choice quiz specifically formulated to market Viagra and to convince the likely consumer that he needs the drug. For example, the first question asks, "Over the past six months: How do you rate your confidence that you could get and keep an erection?" Possible answers are very low, low, moderate, high, and very high. This question plays on a likely consumer's sexual confidence or anxiety, while also making erectile dysfunction seem common. The website informs consumers that "the results will tell you if you have signs of ED (erectile dysfunction)."

The section "Getting a Prescription" features tips on navigating what is assumed to be uncomfortable territory in talking to a doctor about erectile dysfunction. The website tries to normalize and de-stigmatize Viagra use by saying, "And remember, you're not the first one to talk to his doctor about Viagra. Over half of men over 40 have ED to some degree." There are several features of the website that encourage and reward Viagra consumption. Pfizer creates an entire habitus within which an ideal consumer is invited to recognize himself and dwell.[53] As Michele White observes regarding how consumers engage with websites, "Individuals do more than use the Internet and computer; they are instructed to personalize things and follow rules. They are also encouraged to interact, find community, and identify with representations that 'live' within Internet 'space.'"[54] One of the main ways consumers are invited to live within Viagra culture is through active consumption. Value card programs at local grocery stores function in a similar way, in that the Viagra value card gathers consumer demographic data each time they fill a prescription through the "My Value Card Account."[55] Along with consumer information, physician information is also conveyed so that Pfizer sales representatives are able to target more effectively particular doctors as more or less likely to write prescriptions.

Viagra and other erectile dysfunction drugs circulate within and contribute to a contemporary cultural context characterized by the reign of neoliberal political and market practices that "work to construct a 'healthy male citizen'" and "promote individualized responsibility for the management of health and well-being."[56] Not only in terms of sexual health but also in all other areas of corporeal and mental functioning, active consumers have replaced passive patients as idealized agents of their own well-being. Here we see how the logics of neoliberalism are internalized through the processes of medicalization that transform patients into consumer-patients; our daily lives provide endless opportunity for the commodification of health and illness. By "logics of neoliberalism," I refer not only to the ideology that favors unfettered, deregulated markets and dismantled social welfare structures, but also an ideology of the self based on self-reliance, self-sufficiency, and, like Brenda Weber argues in relation to the makeover genre, a production and maintenance of the self as citizen-consumer.[57] Commercials for Viagra and other erectile dysfunction drugs emphasize the post-makeover male body, enhanced and confident, as the result of therapeutic citizenship.

Consequently, in one sense Pfizer's various commercial campaigns have facilitated an open recognition of the failing or inadequacy of middle-aged and old men's sexual performance. Male sexuality is revealed to be, in fact, a performance that is individualized and variable.[58] Male sexual performance that does not live up to hegemonic masculinity's norms is both pathologized and rendered as fragile, constructed, synthesized, and dependent on a little blue pill for support. Yet, in another sense, by foregrounding the vulnerability of male (hetero)sexual performance, ideologies of normative masculinity are all the more entrenched, as Viagra offers a type of guarantee of vital power.[59] The Viagra effect works both ways: while calling attention to the fragility of male sexual performance, here defined rather narrowly and subjectively as an erect penis that is controlled by a man, the commercial discourses surrounding Viagra consumption also reify the penis as a playful tool and men as agents who set the rules of the game. While one level of popular discourse about Viagra, as represented by commercials and Pfizer's official website, seems to both disrupt and consolidate heteronormative male sexual performance, a popular parallel discourse conveyed through jokes, YouTube videos, and assorted parodic texts destabilizes hegemonic ideas about embodied male masculinity and desire. The material and popular culture of Viagra, this chapter argues, incorporates contradictory ideologies of masculinity and sexuality, which facilitate the stabilization of hegemonic masculinity while appearing to destabilize it. In relation to the gendered depiction of a contradictory masculinity, we can also see the ways that the idea of the consumer-patient encompasses dual notions of limited agency and reliance on professional experts. If, through the Viagra case study, hegemonic masculinity is offered up as both fragile and yet ultimately powerful, then the position of the consumer-patient is equally burdened with these apparently contradictory conditions. The fragility of hegemonic masculinity is simultaneously exposed and supported through the medicalization of aging and old men.

As previous chapters demonstrated, television and other media engage the logic of spatial therapeutics, in which structures and bodies are positioned in such a way as to enhance treatment and rehabilitation. The possibilities of television as a therapeutic medium call for an engagement with the limits, or potential ill effects, of such scenarios. At the same time, this positioning, in terms of hospital space, is accompanied by a discourse of therapeutic agency that addresses an ideal, hybrid subject: the consumer-patient. This therapeutic positioning in relation to television, hospital space, and the consumer-patient continues once the individual returns home. While inpatients may be discharged from hospitals, consumer-patients remain subject to other therapeutic discourses and practices in the form of television commercials for prescription drugs, health-oriented reality programs such as *The Dr. Oz Show*

(NBC, 2009–), or through home-based health care. In this case study of two of Pfizer's Viagra campaigns, we can see how direct-to-consumer drug commercials work simultaneously to restore and revise dominant versions of heteronormative masculinity and consistently remind us, as consumers, of the therapeutic framing of everyday life. As Regula Valerie Burri and Joseph Dumit observe, "Life itself has become subject to new modes of intervention and governance which create a new form of genetic and biological citizenship.... Illnesses are 'invented,' and new 'pharmaceutical' ways of thinking emerge."[60] Therapeutic positioning, via spaces such as hospitals or homes, accompanies this new pharmaceutical way of thinking and, together, they encourage us to become increasingly aware of ourselves as consumer-patients. In the case of Viagra, we can see that messages about erectile dysfunction, as a male health issue, are simultaneously informative, entertaining, and constitutive of what Burri and Dumit mean by a pharmaceutical way of thinking.[61] As dynamics that may be resisted in some contexts, recognized and lived through in others, pharmaceutical thinking and spatial therapeutics nonetheless suggest that our ways of engaging with television in the space of the hospital or at home may indeed be therapeutic. This includes the definition of therapeutic to refer to several things, such as a temporary diversion from worry, a feeling of connection to friends and family while one is in the hospital, a sense of agency (however minimal) in relation to one's illness or condition, or a feeling of security and care in one's home. But it is important to emphasize that there is no purely therapeutic encounter with media; there are ways in which television and other media are used to facilitate a therapeutic experience and to restructure our encounters with, for example, hospitalization and what it means to be a patient-consumer. It is this possibility of positioning television as a therapeutic agent, as a healing medium, not simply or uniformly as the source of what ails us, that has animated this book. Yet, in opening the possibility of rethinking how television functions in particular places, and by replacing television in locations such as the de-institutionalized hospital or the medicalized home, we cannot ignore that television, in its entertainment, in its diversion, in its offer of therapeutic agency, is always more than a consoling bedside companion.

# Conclusion
## OUR BODIES, OUR (TV) SELVES

On January, 15, 2008, Oprah Winfrey extended her brand and status as media mogul with a "new multi-platform media venture" called, not ironically, "OWN: The Oprah Winfrey Network." OWN is a joint venture between Discovery Health Channel and Winfrey's Harpo Productions.[1] Harpo is corporate home of the long-running and popular *The Oprah Winfrey Show*. Winfrey's production company creates original television programming, operates the website Oprah.com, publishes the monthly magazine *O: The Oprah Magazine* in a partnership with Hearst Magazines, and broadcasts the Oprah Radio channel on SiriusXM satellite radio.[2]

This mutually beneficial economic partnership between Harpo and Discovery Health gives each media company something that the other lacks.[3] For Harpo, the Discovery Health partnership grants a different kind of cultural legitimacy through Discovery's ties to educational, nonfiction content as well as a huge international audience.[4] Harpo brings to Discovery significant numbers of female viewers in a demographic prized by advertisers. With its emphasis on self-help and self-health, OWN offers Discovery Health a warmer, more familiar—even feminine—style of original programming that will enhance and further entwine the educational and entertainment features of each media company. As Sarah Banet-Weiser argues in relation to the cable network Nickelodeon and its branding strategies, "Contemporary strategies of branding work to commodify an *experience*—not just a product—for audiences."[5]

Corporate executives at Discovery Communications, while not using Banet-Weiser's exact words, have nonetheless articulated a similar understanding of how OWN facilitates an affective circuit within which television viewers and computer users will circulate. As part of the deal, Winfrey enjoys complete editorial control over "programming, branding, and creative vision."[6] Recognizing the need for spreading her own brand of self-help and self-inspiration, Winfrey described OWN as a "natural extension" of Harpo, while Discovery Communications President and CEO David Zaslav emphasized Winfrey's personal commitment to health and the shared goals of multi-platform product and experiential branding: "There is no stronger voice than Oprah Winfrey in engaging, motivating and connecting people to live healthier lives. Oprah has inspired me personally, and through this new venture, Oprah's talent and drive will have a dedicated multimedia platform to empower, engage and connect people on-air and on-line. At Discovery, our goals are to improve the quality of the networks while expanding the reach and success of our web presence. This venture does both, and having Oprah as Chairman and creative leader makes OWN a very unique property in a crowded media landscape."[7] In this case, extending Discovery's brand into health —as represented by Winfrey's emphasis on the health of her audience— allows the media corporation to promote itself as a unique property. It accomplishes this, as the previous two chapters have shown in the case of pharmaceutical corporations, through an apparently altruistic investment in its viewers.

Extending the brand and audience for both Discovery Health and Harpo, OWN centralizes *and* circulates Oprah Winfrey's popularization of medical and health-related expertise. As Discovery Health struggled to maintain a profitable presence in relation to other Discovery Communications networks, this joint venture is expected to be just the prescription for increasing advertising revenue and ratings among some of the most highly prized viewers. OWN creates a brand that espouses the philosophy of "living your best life."[8]

The partnership between Discovery Health and Winfrey suggests that the former, launched on August 12, 1999, needed its own makeover. After almost ten years of providing various kinds of reality-based, health-related programming—from the exploration of medical forensic science with *Dr. G: Medical Examiner*, to transformation programming like *Plastic Surgery: Before and After*, as well as syndicated shows such as *Extreme Makeover*—Discovery Health has conceived of its television programming "with both the TV and Web components in mind, so the two operations can enhance each other."[9] With the marketing slogan "Real stories. Real people. Real medicine," Discovery Health has been a natural home for a host of health-related marketers, including pharmaceutical corporations. In 2001 Discovery Health altered its programming to include more nonfiction programs that gave viewers a sense of "control over their health" in an effort to boost potential distribution over the thirty million household mark (via cable systems)—the threshold that pharmaceutical companies were waiting for the network to cross before buying advertising time.[10]

As Discovery Health shifted toward do-it-yourself health programming and developed its multi-platform approach to health content, in 2006 the network hired the health and pharmaceutical industry leader Leonard J. Tacconi as president. Tacconi was a perfect match for Discovery Health in that he brought years of experience as a former executive director of corporate marketing at Merck, a leading pharmaceutical corporation, as well as having been the North American marketing director for weight-loss and other services at Weight Watchers International. Emphasizing the activity of consumers in relation to their own health, Tacconi described his goal at Discovery Health as one that would increase the network's "position as a trusted partner in providing high-quality information across current and emerging media channels."[11] Representing the merger of pharmaceutical industries (Merck) and consumer empowerment (Weight Watchers), Tacconi's experience was understood as an asset for Discovery Health. This example shows, as the book has elaborated, the web of economic and ideological connection between the corporation and the utilization of the self-health, domestic appeal.

Yet it is clear that while Discovery Health undergoes its own transformation in terms of corporate ownership and programming, viewers also undergo a similar transformation. We are encouraged, more and more, to shape ourselves, quite literally, as healthy subjects and to recognize ourselves as consumer-patients. While it is surely the case that the subject position of the consumer-patient may be resisted, there are profound ways in which we claim it and can make it our own. As Brenda R. Weber demonstrates in her thorough account of the makeover reality television genre, the participants in programs such as *The Swan* or *The Biggest Loser* agree to appear for a variety of reasons and are not simply and in any straightforward way ideological dupes.[12] In relation to the therapeutic aspects of television, I want to stress a similar conviction. Television may indeed position us as consumer-patients, but we may enact this subjectivity while still remaining skeptical of its benefits, resisting its categorization, and adapting its commercial messages to our own needs. The processes of spatial therapeutics and medicalization require some level of participation for them to make sense. What can come from this participation—even if it is critical participation—is a more active way of being a consumer-patient, if we should one day find ourselves in such a position.

Does television make us healthier? This book does not make that claim, but it does prod us to rethink not only our relationship to television, but also our ideas about what it means to be healthy. If we turn off our televisions and avoid pharmaceutical advertising, will our homes and bodies cease to be medicalized? The answer is no. The processes of medicalization and the positioning of individuals as potential patients are ongoing and happening in other social, cultural, economic, and political formations and at the level of public policy and law, as the contentious passage of the Patient Protection and Affordable Care Act in March 2010 exemplifies. Health, in this context, becomes not necessarily something that someone has, but rather something someone should have a legal right to. It is, moreover, a model of health based on keeping the current for-profit features of American health care in place, rather than a full-scale revision of this system with an actual public or national health system.

As for television, the creation of OWN, as a multi-platform, self-health, self-help multimedia entity, makes explicit one of the main ideas developed throughout *Prescription TV*. In all its media incarnations, OWN is emblematic of the transformation of the home into a modern health information center. No longer confined to the medicine cabinet or the doctor's office, consumers now have multi-mediated medical information on a variety of home screens, from television to their computers to their mobile devices. Offered not only information but also in some cases diagnostic tools, consumers have the ability to download expertise that, previously, only physicians or other medical experts had. This is not to say that all health-related information available on television or the Internet is reliable or credible, but then how do we know when to trust our physicians? It is fundamental to recognize that all health information is framed by particular interests. Whether it should be that way is a legitimate question, but it would be naive to say that just because we access information via the media that we should be less trustful of its credibility—as if the medium is, as Marshall McLuhan suggested, the message. Rather, it is just as important to trace the ways that television consistently, through health networks, talk shows, makeover programs, and drug commercials, offers a means of circulating ideas about health, medicalization, and what it means to be a healthy, self-conscious citizen.

As I have shown in *Prescription TV*, mass media are used to make health care facilities such as hospitals seem both modern and more like home. It is also the case that the availability of health content as both education and entertainment, on the Internet and television, medicalizes the modern home as a center for self-diagnosis and treatment. For example, chapter 1 historicized the arrival of mass media in hospital contexts during the First World War. As film began to be used to facilitate soldiers' recovery and rehabilitation, entertainment took on a unique role in the healing of bodies and minds. Hospital administrators, after the war's end, continued to adapt film exhibition in hospitals as a means of deinstitutionalizing modern hospitals, distracting patients from pain, and providing visions of "something better to escape into," as Richard Dyer has said generally of entertainment.[13] As I explained in chapter 1, radio manufacturers identified hospitals as potential markets for mass media entertainment. Radio, first as a privatized listening experience, was sold to hospital administrators and to patients as a way of making hospitals seem modern and more like home. Chapter 2 continued to explore the idea of hospital deinstitutionalization by recounting the material, architectural history of television's installation in the modern, post–Second World War hospital. In the context of the growing privatization of health care, hospital administrators and designers focused on ways to make the hospital a more inviting, personal, therapeutic space. Chapter 3 elaborated on how television manufacturers seized on the idea of the spatial therapeutics of TV and incorporated it into their advertisements. In selling hospitals on the idea of television, manufacturers prescribed how it should be used in the hospital (and by whom). In the process, the concept and image of the patient as consumer began to take shape, and television's medical reach drew closer to home. Chapters 4 and 5 delved deeper into contemporary manifestations of the relationship between health, media, and the consumer-patient through direct-to-consumer pharmaceutical advertising. We saw how television's role in the medical marketplace became even more central as consumer-patients began to take their health care into their own hands and homes. Both physicians and consumer-patients are courted by different forms of advertising—those that prompt physicians to write prescriptions for specific brand-name drugs, and those that urge consumer-patients to talk to their doctor about those drugs. Direct-to-consumer prescription drug advertising has been part of the redefinition and redistribution of medical expertise and authority, even if it is primarily a transformation based on market terms. In this form of media-health entanglement, we see the manifestation of the medicalization of the modern home, and the transformation of patients into consumer-patients. As this book has shown, over the past hundred years mass media have recast entertainment as a prescription for health.

Today television promises multiple ways to reshape not only our bodies, but also our lives. Toward that end, Discovery Health, the Learning Channel, and other cable and broadcast networks offer health and medical programming that emphasizes the ways good health is achieved through the productive labor of viewing other people's physical transformations. As I have explained throughout the book, various interlocking interests and events have worked to produce, through television, the consumer-patient. Yet another way that the subjectivity of the consumer-patient is produced is through the display of self-health on reality television programming. Both reality television and recent consumer-patient advertising for hospitals indicate the extent to which consumer-patients have become the substance of television, exposing bodies for the presumed benefit of others as well as oneself. As Laurie Ouellette, John McMurria, Anna McCarthy, Dana Heller, and Brenda Weber have argued, reality television is chock-full of programs that promise transformation: of home, of bodies, of taste, of lives.[14] McCarthy has also suggested that one of the pleasures viewers have in watching programs that depict suffering, such as *The Biggest Loser* or *Judge Judy*, in which participants are frequently humiliated in the name of justice, is to be found in the mechanisms of "painful civic pedagogy"—which I would expand to *physical* civic pedagogy—"suffused with tears, rage, and insults." McCarthy explains that the reality genre's "affective dimensions might have something new to teach us about the processes of self-organization in which modern subjects find themselves caught."[15]

With the rise of physician- and consumer-directed prescription drug advertising, the worry was that health would become too commercial, mere entertainment, nothing but a vehicle for marketing new products, services, and illnesses. This could certainly be argued to now be the case, as we see that in addition to taking prescription drugs encouraged by advertisements, viewers are also submitting to various surgeries to lose weight or look better (e.g., liposuction, bariatric surgery)—which they have seen depicted on plastic surgery programs such as *The Swan, Extreme Makeover*, and *Dr. 90210*, and dramas like *Nip/Tuck*.[16] Reality television surgery shows range from those that are cosmetically or generally focused—like *Big Medicine* (TLC), *Trauma: Life in the ER* (Discovery Fit and Health), and *Code Blue* (Discovery Fit and Health)—to medical investigation reality shows—like *Dr. G: Medical Examiner* (Discovery Fit and Health), *Diagnosis: Unknown* and *Mystery Diagnosis* (both on Discovery Fit and Health), and *Hopkins* (ABC). What all these programs have in common is the assumption that bodies can be tools of instruction, whether they are living ones undergoing bariatric surgery or dead ones whose autopsies reveal the cause of death.

While these are reality-based diagnostic/investigative medical programs, they have their fictional counterparts in the forensic gore/reveal of *Bones* (Fox), *CSI* (CBS), and *Law and Order: SVU* (NBC), and the disease as mystery in *House, M.D.* (Fox). Each of these fictional programs spends time in the laboratory, in the morgue, and at the patient's bedside. The doctors as detectives and coroners as crime solvers peer through microscopes and collect blood splatter samples, as the camera takes the point of view of either the murder weapon or the diagnostic probe, flying through blood vessels and permeating internal organs. Not only has medicine become entertainment, the patient has become television.

With reality programs such as NBC's *The Biggest Loser*, moreover, contestants are represented as heroic as they endure all manner of activities, including each episode's revealing weigh-in. In TLC's *Honey, We're Killing the Kids*, a white female nutritional and diet expert enters working- and middle-class homes, frequently of people of color, and instructs the parents on how to change from unhealthy to healthy eating habits. This program urges conformity to normative body size and nutritional conduct in order to position self-regulating subjects.[17] In contrast, pharmaceutical advertisements for Viagra and Flomax do not represent iconography associated with working-class culture; instead, they show actors in posh surroundings such as vacation hot tubs, pristine golf courses, and luxurious yachts. In other words, rarely are plumbers or male greeters at Home Depot featured in commercials for prescription drugs.

Contestants on shows like *The Biggest Loser* become ordinary heroes and temporary celebrities for their ability to transform their own bodies. All one needs to do to become a more productive citizen is to size down and, consequently, measure up to a different socioeconomic position—to become a better, self-regulating citizen by, in the case of weight loss, becoming, literally, less of one. Actual disparities seem inconsequential if one can maintain one's health by talking to a doctor about a new prescription drug. It seems that it is the responsibility of the consumer-patient to use television to receive basic health care.

By no means do I disparage the labor, physical and mental, involved in body-focused makeover reality programs. As McCarthy observes, "To see reality television as merely trivial entertainment is to avoid recognizing the degree to which the genre is preoccupied with the government of the self, and how, in that capacity, it demarcates a zone for the production of everyday discourses of citizenship."[18] On the one hand, however, I wonder if health-related entertainment, as well as the overall medicalization of everyday life, may work as alibis for the state's conditional regard for the health and well-being of the least privileged of its citizens. What happens to the people who did not make it onto *The Biggest Loser* or *Extreme Makeover*? Are there affordable, accessible support services for people who seek surgical or other modes of weight loss (in addition to diet and exercise), or who are in need of dental care? Do we have to be on TV in order to receive basic medical care?[19] If so, what is produced through the labor of becoming a televised patient?[20]

A second powerful television example of the ways that consumer-patients are *on the screen* at the same time as they are in front of it as viewers is the use of actual patients in commercials produced for hospitals and as informational videos for specific kinds of surgery. The spectacularization of the consumer-patient is the logical response to the commodification of health. No longer merely consumer-patients in hospitals or medical centers, we have *become* television, or the material of television itself. For instance, two 2009 articles in the *New York Times* provide proof of this newest twist in the category of the consumer-patient. One article profiles Akron Children's Hospital in Ohio, which produced its own television commercial. Yet it did not feature the hospital's state-of-the-art medical technology, physicians, nurses, or staff.

Rather, the hospital got its message across using a patient: an unscripted commercial featuring Austin, a fourteen-year-old boy diagnosed with cancer and undergoing chemotherapy. The commercial focuses on Austin as he walks through hospital corridors and sits in a chair, discussing his diagnosis and treatment. Physicians and nurses never appear, nor does any kind of "direct reference" to the hospital. Only at the end of the commercial do we see the hospital's website URL appear on the screen.

Austin's spot is one of several that the hospital is running in its regional market. Unlike other commercials and advertisements for hospitals, these series of spots include "patients in the throes of crises, with no inkling of their outcomes." Contrary to typical testimonial advertising, where the positive outcome of a situation is obvious, these in-the-middle-of-treatment commercials do not give viewers the comfort of seeing a success story. Instead, according to Jim Sollisch, one of the creative directors at the Marcus Thomas advertising agency in Cleveland, these commercials featuring patients going through their illness allow for the spot itself to "reflect the inherent drama in the situation."[21]

The hospital and its marketing agency seem aware of the exploitative aspects of this practice; in fact, they see this as precisely one of the strengths of such an approach. Sollisch claims that the campaign, "aimed at mothers ages 18–49, reflects the spirit of YouTube and Facebook, where nonactors are the stars, and spontaneity trumps scripted messages."[22] Embracing the amateur and the unscripted format, this example of the spectacularization of the consumer-patient foregrounds the ways that our bodies, our lives, and our health are used as commercial product for the creation of health care that puts us first. The commercial assumes that consumer-patients, moreover, have the right to choose a hospital, that selecting a hospital for one's care is like selecting any other kind of service. These commercials demonstrate the ordinariness of illness, while they also narrowcast their message to those viewers who have the means to make such a treatment choice in the first place.

In another example of how consumer-patients literally become television, Methodist University Hospital in Memphis circulated a video webcast of Shila Renee Mullins's "awake craniotomy, in which the patient remains conscious and talking while surgeons prod and cut inside her brain." Mullins's surgery was also promoted on television infomercials and newspaper advertisements "featuring a photograph of a beautiful model, not Ms. Mullins." It is interesting that the promotional materials featured a model rather that a photograph of the patient herself when other parts of her seemed perfectly fine for display. A health care marketing consultant, Tony Cotrupi, commented that patients "used to go like sheep wherever the doctor sent us. . . . But now, you have the curious consumer and hospitals are doing all they can to open up the kimono."[23] While I hesitate to believe that hospitals are indeed "doing all they can to open up the kimono"—a strangely sexualized and exoticized reference to describe what I would call an example of the deinstitutionalization of modern hospitals—it is nonetheless instructive that these two promotional texts are marketing their health care through consumer-patients. Some hospitals have even encouraged their consumer-patients to blog about their procedures, including Genesis Health System in Davenport, Iowa, which features blogs about bariatric surgery. Our bodies and our illnesses, once considered private, or at least only visible to medical professionals, are now fodder for television infomercials, webcasts, Twitter messages, and blogs. Yet consumer-patients are not coerced into participating; rather, they seem proud to be providing information for other potential consumer-patients, demystifying what could be seen as complicated and frightening procedures. At any rate, these examples of consumer-patient television, from reality programs to commercials for hospitals, further establish the ways that the transformation of the patient to the consumer has been accomplished through television.

From film to commercials for prescription drugs to self-help medical and health websites such as PatientsLikeMe.com (which includes the pharmaceutical manufacturer Novartis as one of its corporate partners), the prognosis for health and contemporary media is the production of more nonfiction, reality-based programming in which pedagogies of normative, healthy citizenship are taught. As a means to address an increasingly narrow slice of the consumerist pie, health-related media will continue to refine their focus to ever more specific and affluent audiences: those with the ability to pay for advertised products and services. Yet it may be the case that, as the requirements of the 2010 Patient Protection and Affordable Care Act begin to affect the health insurance market, television extends its focus to account for the millions of new consumer-patients who will be required to purchase health coverage.

I began this book by telling a personal story about my father and me watching television together while he was in the hospital. I conclude this book by telling another personal story, this one about my mother, television, the Internet, and the medicalization of home. My eighty-six-year-old mother lives in Denton, Texas, and had, until the second presidential term of George W. Bush, been a lifelong Republican. During Barack Obama's campaign, however, my mother volunteered at her local, very small, Democratic Party headquarters. She was so active in her advocacy —with health care, the economy, and the wars being her top issues— that the Obama campaign sent her special recognition.

A few months ago, my mother, who has always been an avid reader and critical television watcher, decided that she needed to get a computer. She wanted a laptop. She signed up for computer classes at the local public library and hired a tutor to help her at home. I was delighted to receive my first e-mail message from her. One of the main reasons my mother wanted to get a computer, apart from its obvious benefits to her research as a self-taught historian and newspaper columnist, was that she could access more information about health and medical care for senior adults. With the computer, my mother has learned that she is connected to many other individuals who are dealing with some of the same health issues that affect her. She is learning about advocacy groups, medical research, and self-care. In short, my mother is an active consumer-patient, wary of commercial websites and prescription drug commercials, but also ready to admit that she benefits from the drugs advertised on the websites she visits. My mother's eyesight is failing, slowly, so the computer allows her to magnify images and words and to continue to read about treatments and physicians, and to communicate with other people who have the same illnesses. My mother lives alone, but she tells me that she feels connected to the twenty-first century. She is amazed by the fact that she does not have to leave her home to get credible medical information. She exchanges e-mails with her current physician's assistant, who keeps up with patients online.

Recently my mother was diagnosed with a rare illness that neither of us nor any of our friends or family had ever heard of. Her previous personal physician, a geriatric specialist, had apparently not done a thorough job of explaining this condition to my mother. So, while she was on her home computer, she called me and told me to get on mine. Together, as we tried to keep our emotions from getting the best of us, we read information from the Mayo Clinic and the National Institutes of Health websites. In addition, my mother receives regular e-mails from her physician and physician's assistant via their smart phones. The phenomenon my mother is experiencing, called "aging in place," is part of the contemporary medicalization of the home. Aging in place assumes that individuals, if given a choice, would prefer to stay in their own homes, to age in place, rather than have to leave their homes to enter a medical care facility. It is a process of medicalization that relies in part on media access, and which is being facilitated, at a national and governmental level, through the development of public policies such as those advocated in the March 2010 report *The National Broadband Plan: Connecting America*, compiled by the Federal Communications Commission. This national plan, according to *Wired* magazine, is "a sort of Declaration of the Internet that seeks to ensure that a fast broadband connection is just as much an unalienable right as life, liberty, and the pursuit of happiness."[24]

Home health care, for people living in rural areas or people who, like my mother, have a difficult time getting to the physician, is an important part of the plan. The FCC indicates how broadband service facilitates many things, including processes of home medicalization. One of the goals of this plan is to "reform laws, policies, standards, and incentives to maximize the benefits of broadband in sectors government influences greatly, such as public education, health care, and government operation."[25] In April 2010 the U.S. Senate Special Committee on Aging convened a hearing called "The National Broadband Plan and Bringing Health Care Technology Home." Among the various senators representing rural states such as Maine were representatives from the FCC, organizations such as the American Association of Homes and Services for the Aging, and physicians who practice telemedicine, or distance medicine that involves the use of computer technology to monitor patients.[26] The assumptions that structured the hearing and the National Broadband Plan, as they pertain to health, are that home is and should be medicalized via the Internet, and that it is in the best interest of consumer-patients to participate in this mode of health monitoring, surveillance, and care. With the rise of "e-care," which conflates media and health, not only does the home become medicalized, but consumer-patients participate in this process as ideal citizen patients and as key components of the nation's vision of itself as a caring, *connected* America.

My mother's experience as a contemporary health and media consumer aging in place shows that there are many ways that homes become medicalized and that we live as consumer-patients. In relation to my father and my mother, television and the Internet have indeed been therapeutic, but in very different kinds of ways. For my father, television was a comfort and a distraction while he was in the hospital. For my mother, television and the Internet at home have helped her feel connected to me and engaged with different kinds of communities. It is this possibility of connections offered through film, radio, and television in hospitals and at home—to information, to entertainment, to one another—that is perhaps the most therapeutic tonic of them all.

# Notes

## INTRODUCTION

1 *Deinstitutionalization*, as I am using it, refers to the creation of a new perception of the modern hospital. But the term also has a different, very specific meaning that refers to public health policies, implemented at the beginning of the 1960s, that facilitated new practices and procedures in the admission and release of patients in mental hospitals. Deinstitutionalization, as it has been commonly understood and as it applies to the United States, took its contemporary form in the 1960s as a reform movement aimed at mental health policies and practices. Designed to revise the ways that mental health and disability were legally defined (and treatment was determined), policies directed toward deinstitutionalization favored outpatient and community release of individuals from hospitalization. Yet the type of deinstitutionalization I refer to has more to do with efforts by the hospital industry to redefine the negative connotations of the institutional aspects of hospitals. For more information on the history of deinstitutionalization as a public health policy that was originally conceived as a reform movement, but which has had negative consequences for patient care, see Torrey, *Out of the Shadows*; Porter, *Madness*; and Rosenberg, *The Care of Strangers*. For a perspective on deinstitutionalization that relates more to my use of the term, which I will elaborate later in the introduction, see Verderber and Fine, *Health Care Architecture in an Era of Radical Transformation*.

2 See Crawford, "Health as a Meaningful Social Practice."

3 See Weber, *Makeover TV*; Ouellette and Hay, *Better Living through Reality TV*.

4 Even before watchdog groups and mass communication researchers began

to express concern over the effects of television on society, previous studies —such as eight books published by the Committee on Educational Research of the Payne Fund—focused on film and radio and represented mass media as detrimental to the public interest. See Draper, "Controversy Has Probably Destroyed Forever the Context," for a history of censorship and decency in a case study of the film *The Miracle* (1948). Draper describes the list of books published by the Payne Fund and its concern for the relation between media and the public good.

5  Emblematic of such criticisms of television is a recent 2008 study conducted by the entrepreneur and self-proclaimed media expert James Steyer, founder of the media advocacy or watchdog group Common Sense Media, in collaboration with the Department of Clinical Bioethics at the National Institutes of Health. The published findings, "Media + Child and Adolescent Health: A Systematic Review," consisted of a selected review of 173 quantitative studies of media exposure in relation to child or adolescent health in seven key areas: childhood obesity, tobacco use, drug use, alcohol use, low academic achievement, sexual behavior, and attention deficit disorder with hyperactivity. Culled from existing quantitative studies from 1980 to 2008 and "using appropriate database-specific search terms for media as well as the health outcomes of interest," the review team, consisting of five medical doctors, found that in "80 percent of the studies, greater media exposure is associated with negative health outcomes for children and adolescents." See Common Sense Media, "Media + Child and Adolescent Health: A Systematic Review," November 2008, http://www.commonsensemedia .org/. Still, after decades of studying the effects of television and children, the best that can be determined is that there is an *association* among these negative traits, and each new study can only suggest that television is the culprit. While other media scholars and other researchers, including physicians and public health advocates, have produced thoughtful counterarguments to the negative-effects approach, the equation of television plus children equals bad habits or bad health continues to dominate popular discourse and public policy.

6  This has been well documented by Lynn Spigel in *Make Room for TV*.

7  It is important to examine the assumptions about television to understand how these apparently diametrically opposed discourses can exist at the same time.

8  Seiter, *Television and New Media Audiences*, 117.

9  See Serlin, "Performing Live Surgery on Television and the Internet since 1945."

10 Gamson, *Freaks Talk Back*; White, *Tele-Advising*; Weber, *Makeover TV*; Shattuc, *The Talking Cure*.

11 Friedman, "Introduction," 7.

12 Thompson, *Television's Second Golden Age*; Turow, *Playing Doctor*.

13 See McCarthy, *Ambient TV*; Riggs, *Mature Audiences*; Treichler, Cart-

wright, and Penley, eds., *The Visible Woman*; Cartwright, *Screening the Body*; Terry and Calvert, eds., *Processed Lives*; Balsamo, *Technologies of the Gendered Body*; and Price and Shildrick, eds., *Vital Signs*.

14  See Gilman's *Disease and Representation* and *Picturing Health and Illness*; Kraut, *Silent Travelers*; and Leavitt, *Typhoid Mary*.

15  See Crimp, ed., *AIDS*; Patton, *Inventing AIDS*; Erni, *Unstable Frontiers*; Waldby, *AIDS and the Body Politic*; Watney, *Policing Desire*; Treichler, *How to Have Theory in an Epidemic*.

16  These studies may be found in various disciplines or academic fields, such as health communication. See, for example, Jackson and Duffy, *Health Communication Research*; Atkin and Wallack, eds., *Communication and Public Health*; and Lammers and Geist, "The Transformation of Caring in the Light and Shadow of 'Managed Care.'"

17  McCarthy, *Ambient Television*, 119.

18  This is not to say that different forms of consumption have not been examined in relation to various practices and objects. The dominant paradigm within consumer culture studies privileges retail shopping and the female consumer. Moreover, within the interdisciplinary field of the medical humanities, television has most often been examined through textual analysis that focuses on the image of the physician. In fact, there is a significant body of work on the history of the representation of the television doctor, as Joseph Turow and others point out, from the early 1950s to the 2000s (with the complicated image of the doctor as hero in *House, M.D.*). More often than not, medical humanities scholarship focuses more on interpreting media portrayals of doctors rather than asking questions about why doctors are being portrayed on television in the first place. Additionally, the spaces within which television is watched are rarely examined as contributing to how medical messages are received and understood.

19  Foucault, *The Care of the Self*.

20  Weber, *Makeover TV*.

21  Ibid., 39.

22  See McCarthy's chapter "Television while You Wait," from *Ambient Television*, 195–223. CBS provides content for Healium Network through original and existing programming. CBS Press Express, "CBS to Provide Exclusive Branded Content for the Healium (TM) Waiting Room Network," CBS press release, July 19, 2007, www.cbspressexpress.com/cbs-sports/releases/view?id=16382.

23  Crawford, "Health as a Meaningful Social Practice," 415.

24  Williams, *Keywords*, 23.

25  Tiefer, "The Medicalization of Impotence," 363.

26  Clarke et al., "Biomedicalization"; Treichler, Cartwright, and Penley, *The Visible Woman*; Treichler, *How to Have Theory*; Cartwright, *Screening the Body* and "Rural Telemedicine and the Globalization of U.S. Health Care"; Tiefer, "The Medicalization of Impotence," *Sex Is Not a Natural Act*, and "The Viagra Phenomenon"; Waldby, *AIDS and Body Politic*.

27  Clarke et al., "Biomedicalization," 163.
28  Ibid., 166.
29  Tomes, "Patients or Health-Care Consumers?," 84.
30  Ibid., 85, 99.
31  George Annas quoted in ibid., 83.
32  President Barack Obama, on March 23, 2010, signed the Patient Protection and Affordable Care Act into law, after months of heated partisan arguments and with television entering the fray as a key source of competing interpretations of the legislation and its proposed effects. This law promises to be the most significant health care legislation since Medicare was enacted in 1965 during the Lyndon B. Johnson administration and as part of the Great Society programs. President Obama campaigned on, among other things, health care reform, and according to the U.S. Census Bureau, there were 46.3 million uninsured individuals in the United States in 2008, an increase from the 2007 figure of 45.7 million. While this figure represents individuals without health insurance, it does not consider individuals without health care. As has been explained by supporters of the Obama administration's approach to health care reform, having health insurance does not guarantee the receipt of health care services. Denial of coverage, caps on reimbursements, limits on lifetime coverage, and lack of portability often work to deny necessary procedures to individuals who already have health insurance. The market-based model, which has facilitated insurance oligopolies in the United States, may be mitigated, but not disassembled, by the 2010 health care legislation. As opposed to Medicare, however, which was constructed in a New Deal orientation, Obama's legislation is conservative, "building on a Republican rather than a New Deal philosophy," according to Robert Reich. Yet the 2010 health care legislation does have significant consequences, at least politically and hopefully economically, because it "reasserts that government can provide a major solution" to social issues such as lack of health care. It keeps in place, however, the profit-based structures of the current medical marketplace and ensures that we will continue to function as consumer-patients within it. See Robert Reich, "The Final Health Care Vote and What It Really Means," March 21, 2010, http://robertreich.org/. See also Reid, *The Healing of America*.
33  Tomes, "Patients or Health-Care Consumers?," 106
34  Included in Discovery's cable television collection are the following networks: Animal Planet, Discovery Channel, Discovery Fit and Health, Discovery Kids, Military Channel, OWN: The Oprah Winfrey Network, Science Channel, and TLC.
35  There are notable studies of television outside and in addition to domestic space. See Couldry and McCarthy, eds., *MediaSpace*.
36  Lisa Cartwright, along with other media scholars and historians, has documented the role of film in medical science and in public health campaigns. Scholarly attention has tended to focus on the *content* of medical images

rather than the *context* within which they were produced or received. When studies have considered the *context* for films with an explicit health or medical focus, as in public hygiene or breast cancer education films, they have not examined what purpose film and other media serve within a hospital or clinical space. Two anthologies that come the closest to exploring the history of the uses of media within clinical contexts are Cartwright, *Screening the Body*; Reagan, Tomes, and Treichler, eds., *Medicine's Moving Pictures*; and Serlin, ed., *Imagining Illness*.

37   Acland, "Take Two," 198.

### 1: CONVALESCENT COMPANIONS

1   Film and television as medical instruction media within clinical contexts were preceded by photography, beginning in the mid-nineteenth century. With the work of G. B. Duchenne de Boulogne, a founder of the field of neurology and Jean-Martin Charcot's teacher, photography was used to attempt to represent and classify various types of neurological and mental disorders. The focus, as Tom Gunning has shown, was on the subject's face as the external sign of internal meaning. It was with Charcot that photography was incorporated into a specific hospital context. With the development of motion pictures a few decades later, this new medium was also put to use. Previous experiments with photography motion studies, such as those of Eadweard Muybridge and Etienne Jules-Marey, had been applied to a medical context that focused on images of patients produced for the education of medical students, elite members of society, and other invited guests. As early as 1892, Georges Demeny, Marey's assistant, adapted chronophotographic strips to make a phenakistoscope of himself mouthing phrases as tools for teaching deaf people to lip-read. This early history of photography and motion pictures for the documentation of patients' symptoms, clinical observation, and medical education framed the context for the eventual adoption of closed-circuit television in hospitals during the late 1940s. The idea that unites these three media forms is that each one can capture and convey accuracy, intimacy, and, especially with television, liveness. See Cartwright, *Screening the Body*; Gilman, *Disease and Representation*; Dumit, *Picturing Personhood*; and Gunning, "In Your Face."

2   The radio historian Susan Douglas has documented the public debates surrounding radio in its early years, and the role of jazz music as potentially harmful. She has also noted that "most modes of listening generate a strong sense of belonging. Even as mere background noise, radio provides people with a sense of security that silence does not, which is why they actively turn to it, even if they aren't actively listening." This seems especially applicable to hospitalization, when patients are cut off from the outside world. See Douglas, *Listening In*, 8.

3   Elizabeth Richey Dessez, "How the Motion Picture Fits into the Hospital Scheme," *The Modern Hospital* 30, no. 4 (1928): 148–50.

4   The hospital historian Charles Rosenberg explains that in "mid-nineteenth-century America it was well understood that, aside from an occasional emergency, none but the truly indigent would enter a hospital; the working poor preferred to pay a local practitioner if they could or tolerate a dispensary physician's casual visits. Only when length or severity of sickness over-taxed family resources would they consider hospital care" (*The Care of Strangers*, 237).

5   As Lynn Spigel has noted, "Television was debated throughout numerous fields of knowledge, including architecture, interior design, pedagogy, medicine, social science, psychoanalysis, and others. By looking at the popular magazines as discursive sites, we can better account for the diverse number and kinds of meanings attached to television during the period of its installation" (*Make Room for TV*, 8). I would add that this way of analyzing magazines as discursive sites applies equally to professional and trade magazines, and that we can look to them for key meanings about earlier media such as film and radio.

6   Ibid.

7   Ibid., 245.

8   See, for example, Eugene R. Kelly, "Norfolk County Hospital—A Home-Like Institution," *The Modern Hospital* 15, no. 2 (August 1920): 81–84.

9   The phrase "care of strangers" comes from the title of Rosenberg's *The Care of Strangers*.

10  For example, in "How to Select Hospital Furniture," Duane Wanamaker, writing in 1921, observes that "the old-fashioned, gloomy, badly furnished and depressing hospital is rapidly disappearing and the modern hospital is more like a first-class hotel than anything else." At the same time as there seems to have been an emphasis on decorating hospitals to resemble hotels, however, just as much emphasis was placed on creating a homelike atmosphere. See Duane Wanamaker, "How to Select Hospital Furniture," *The Modern Hospital* 17, no. 5 (1921): 433. *The Modern Hospital* began publication in 1913 and continues today under the name *Modern Healthcare*. Spanning almost a century, this professional publication offers rich commentary on everything related to hospital management, from dietary issues for patients to recommendations about how to incorporate media into the existing structures of hospitals.

11  Mrs. Foster was the editor for the CMPB, while her husband set up the infrastructure for the distribution of film to the troops in England and France. She was the one who viewed films and decided which ones were suitable for soldiers. Writing after the war, Mrs. Foster noted that "just as entertainment, the movie contributes pep and ginger and nothing in the wine shops can compare with it as medicine for boys on the march" ("Millions of Feet of Movie Films for Soldiers," *New York Times*, May 5, 1918).

12  Ibid.

13  Ibid.

14   "Moving Pictures Displayed on Camp Hospital Ceilings," *The Modern Hospital* 11, no. 3 (1918): 177.
15   *The Moving Picture World* documents that in 1920, George Eastman had "done another big thing! This time the 'father of the motion picture industry' has given $4,000,000 in conjunction with $5,000,000 from the General Education Board to found a medical school and hospital at the University of Rochester. . . . This latest gift on the part of Mr. Eastman, head of the Eastman Kodak Co., brings the total of his benefactions up to more than $31,000,000." Not only was Eastman instrumental in the founding of the University of Rochester's medical and dental schools, by 1928, through a variety of influences within the industry he organized Eastman Teaching Films Inc., which produced films for public schools and medical schools. See Slide, *Before Video*, 40–42. *The Moving Picture World* was published from 1907 to 1927 and promoted itself as "the official organ of the Moving Picture Exhibitors." As such, it is significant not only for its wealth of information about the industrial and economic aspects of the motion picture industry, but for its social and cultural commentary on topics as diverse as the regulation of film decency to public hygiene and the role of the motion picture industry in serving the needs of the nation during the First World War.
16   The Eastman Kodak Company, beginning in the 1920s, had its own medical division that published books explaining how to use radiography and how such imaging technologies could be applied in medicine and dentistry, as well as instructional pamphlets about how photography could be used by medical professionals in clinical contexts. See, for example, *X-Rays*, 1926; *X-Rays in Medicine and Surgery*, 1926; *Clinical Photography as Applied to the Practice of Medicine and Surgery*, 1932 (all distributed by the Eastman Kodak Company Medical Division).
17   "Motion Pictures in the Hospital," *The Modern Hospital* 15, no. 6 (1920): 470.
18   Ibid., 471. Interestingly, while film spectatorship was understood as easing the pain of patients in hospitals, this was precisely one of the reasons that film exhibition was controversial for prisoners. As a source of pleasure, film exhibition was understood as giving convicts a respite from their otherwise-difficult daily lives.
19   Ibid.
20   Indeed, conventional ways of approaching the topics of film spectatorship and spectators are based on a very particular understanding of text and context delimited to, for the most part, spectators sitting within a space, frequently a movie theater or some other space specifically constructed for watching film. While the historians of itinerant and early film exhibition have shown that experiences of the movies have always involved different kinds of spaces (and how these non-theatrical spaces shape spectatorship), the restriction of film studies to typical theatrical spaces has remained strong. For excellent scholarly work that widens this field of vision in rela-

tion to film exhibition and spectatorship history, see Allen and Gomery, *Film History*; DeCordova, *Picture Personalities*; Gomery, *Shared Pleasures*; Musser, *High-Class Moving Pictures*; Peiss, *Cheap Amusements*; Singer, *Melodrama and Modernity*; Staiger, *Interpreting Films*.

21  I am not assuming that film spectators in movie theaters are always healthy, however defined. What I want to point out is that our experience of film, radio, or television, no matter where we watch or listen, is always context specific, part of which includes our physical and mental states as well as the *place* within which we watch and listen.

22  Dessez, "How the Motion Picture Fits into the Hospital Scheme," 148–50.

23  See Moran, *There's No Place Like Home Video*; and Zimmerman, *Reel Families*.

24  This advertisement, one of the earliest specifically acknowledging the hospital as a site for film exhibition and produced by the Eastman Kodak Company's Medical Division, appeared in *The Modern Hospital*, 30, no. 1 (1928): 161.

25  This advertisement shows the therapeutic benefits of private film screening. All equipment is provided by Eastman Kodak Company Medical Division. It appeared in *The Modern Hospital* 32, no. 2 (1930): 125.

26  Dessez, "How the Motion Picture Fits into the Hospital Scheme," 150.

27  See Jowett, "A Capacity for Evil," 19, 28.

28  Many movie exhibitors in the United States responded to the 1918 influenza pandemic by voluntarily closing their theaters out of fear of contagion, while others had their venues forcibly closed by public health officials. See Ostherr, *Cinematic Prophylaxis*.

29  Ibid.

30  "The Plugs Are Busy," *Hygeia* 1, no. 5 (1923): 323. *Hygeia's* articles regarding the use of media in hospitals show the ways that professional associations like the American Medical Association attempted to present the hospital as, on the one hand, a familiar and homelike place, and on the other hand, a sign of technological achievement and modernity.

31  Ibid.

32  Sterne, *The Audible Past*, 160–62.

33  Hilmes, *Radio Voices*, 1.

34  Ibid., 6.

35  Ibid., 6–7.

36  Inez Pugh, "7,276 Head Sets in U.S. Hospitals," *Hospital Management* 29, no. 4 (1925): 51.

37  Ibid., 58.

38  Dr. Brinkley's problem with credibility extended beyond the controversy over his medical training to include his goat-gland transplant procedures that promised to restore men's sexual vitality. Although he enjoyed popularity not only as a medical adviser but also as a cultural commentator, other medical professionals considered him a quack and a threat to the medical

establishment. Brinkley is perhaps best known for the 1938 libel lawsuit he brought against Morris Fishbein, the editor of *JAMA*.

39   See Lee, *The Bizarre Careers of John R. Brinkley*, 63–64; and Brock, *Charlatan*.
40   "Doctors Are Preferred Prospects," *Radio Retailing* 1, no. 3 (1925): 256–57. *Radio Retailing* (published from 1925 to 1942) was a trade publication directed to wholesale and retail sellers of radio, but also contained information about new contexts within which the new medium might be used, such as hospitals and physicians' waiting rooms.
41   Ibid., 256.
42   Ibid., 257.
43   "Hospital Radio—A Worthy Philanthropy and a New Market for the Dealer," *Radio Retailing* 1, no. 1 (1925): 51.
44   This Powerizer Sound System advertisement appeared in *The Modern Hospital* 34, no. 4 (1930): 152.
45   This advertisement is from *The Modern Hospital* 37, no. 6 (1931): 59.
46   "Is Yours a Cheerful Hospital" appeared in *Hospital Management*, August 1935, 7.
47   First made available in 1931 for in-hospital patient use in England, the radio pillow consisted of a pillow that was "wired for reception." For hospitals that did not have loudspeakers or for patients who found head sets too uncomfortable, the radio pillow was just the answer. By February 1932, the radio pillow had been adopted by the U.S. Department of War for installment in 105 army hospitals "located throughout the U.S., Panama, Hawaii, Puerto Rico, and the Philippine Islands." See "Radio Pillows for 105 Army Hospitals," *The Modern Hospital* 38, no. 2 (1932): 97.
48   *Hospital Management* 19, no. 1 (1925): 78.
49   *Hospital Management* 19, no. 15 (1925): 89.
50   *The Modern Hospital* 3, no. 6 (1929): 125.

## 2: TELEVISION GOES TO THE MODERN HOSPITAL

1   The aesthetic move to deinstitutionalize the appearance of the hospital coincided with pilot programs at various municipal hospitals for the study of home care. See, for example, Marcus D. Kogel and Alexander Kruger, "New York City's Long-Range Program for Extending Hospital Care into the Home," *Hospitals*, February 1950, 35.
2   Spigel, *Make Room for TV*. See also McCarthy, *Ambient Television*. Interestingly, in McCarthy's study of TV outside the home, she discusses uses of television in department stores. According to McCarthy, pre–Second World War architects and designers understood the department store as a "machine for selling," which led them to "refashion the postwar store as an ever more concentrated, systematic structure of physical and visual persuasion" (74). The distinction between retail and medical spaces obscures the

merchandising aspects that each share, as well as the extent to which the clinical features of health care facilities increasingly look more like domestic residences or even hotels. Television has, depending on the particular kind of facility, come to be recognized as yet another medical machine taking its place among an array of technological gadgets and diagnostic imaging devices.

3  Spigel, *Make Room for TV*, 5.
4  In the 1950s, closed-circuit television (CCTV) was used in hospitals for patient monitoring. It was also possible, using CCTV, for patients to view the nurse when using the nurse-call system. For either use, a television monitor in the patient's room would be connected to a central television monitor at the nurses' station, allowing both patients and nurses the possibility of a visual connection. See Letourneau and Hamrick, "The Use of Television in Hospitals," 52–54.
5  Stevens, *In Sickness and in Wealth*, 10.
6  Verderber and Fine, *Health Care Architecture in an Era of Radical Transformation*, 20.
7  See Adams, *Medicine by Design*; Upton, *Architecture in the United States*; Thompson and Goldin, *The Hospital*; and Risse, *Mending Bodies, Saving Souls*.
8  Adams, *Medicine by Design*, xxi.
9  Ibid.
10  Ibid.
11  Grossberg, "The In-Difference of Television," 34–35.
12  Verderber and Fine, *Health Care Architecture in an Era of Radical Transformation*, 13. The French term *monobloc* designates the vertical hospital structure whereby a "steel skeleton frame and the elevator make it possible to fit scattered elements into a single mass." For more information on the vertical monobloc, see Rosenfield and Rosenfield, *Hospital Architecture and Beyond*, 37–38.
13  Verderber and Fine, *Health Care Architecture in an Era of Radical Transformation*, 13.
14  Lynaugh and Brush, *American Nursing*, 3.
15  As alternatives to vertical hospitals in urban centers, where land costs were prohibitive, smaller hospitals in the newly constructed suburbs were able to experiment more with architectural design. In addition, given that many of these suburban hospitals were funded privately by a group of investors and by private, tax-deductible contributions, they were able to design and construct buildings that, in a sense, were more representative of the community. Some of these alternatives to the monobloc hospital included the radial (Scott and White Memorial Hospital, Temple, Texas, 1964); the sawtooth (Mary's Help Hospital, Daly City, California, 1964–66); and the triangle (Lane Pavilion of Point Pleasant Hospital, New Jersey, 1964). By the early 1960s, hospital architecture shifted to include designs that would emphasize revised conceptions of efficiency and patient care.

16  Verderber and Fine, *Health Care Architecture in an Era of Radical Transformation*, 21.
17  Richard Neutra, "What Architects Should Know about Patients," *The Modern Hospital* 95, no. 4 (1960): 93, 144.
18  This approach to the issue of health care architecture—in terms of both economics and aesthetics—has also been addressed within the industry of health facilities design. In addition to hospital trade publications such as *The Modern Hospital*, architecture journals such as *Progressive Architect* have, since the 1960s, focused attention on the dynamic relations between building design and health.
19  Verderber and Fine, *Health Care Architecture in an Era of Radical Transformation*, 208.
20  Ibid., 217.
21  *The Modern Hospital* addressed the extent to which hospitals in the United States were entering the Space Age. This language reflected the transition from the New Deal to New Frontier approaches to technological innovations and implementation of social welfare programs.
22  Verderber and Reuman, "Windows, Views, and Health Status in Hospital Therapeutic Environments."
23  Spigel, *Make Room for TV*, 102.
24  There are several ways that the television can be installed in patient rooms. These include wall in-set units, ceiling or wall suspension, and retractable over-bed arm systems. Each type of television installation has its positive and negative aspects. It is, however, interesting to see the extent to which television installation in the institutional space parallels or departs from domestic design technology.
25  See Ulrich's "A Theory of Supportive Design for Healthcare Facilities" and "Biophilic Theory and Research for Healthcare Design." One aspect of supportive design has to do with the incorporation of nature into the built environment. This is referred to as biophilic design and has been used, along with the incorporation of art, music, and color, to create therapeutic spaces in medical contexts.
26  Indeed, some hospital cable television providers have incorporated theories of supportive design (specifically biophilic or nature programming) into their original productions. Hospitals that subscribe to the Healium Network, for example, may offer patients programs that feature images of nature and animals accompanied by soothing music. Even hotels such as the Westin chain offer guests TV programming, along with the Nintendo Wii video game console for exercise, that uses nature and guided mediation programs to create an atmosphere promoting wellness or feelings of relaxation and calm. See "Philips Partners with Westin Hotels and Resorts to Combat Jetlag," September 3, 2008, http://www.newscenter.philips.com/. See also "Westin Hotels Want to Play . . . Westin Announces Industry-First Partnership with Nintendo," May 1, 2008, http://www.nintendo.com/. I

thank Diane Negra for calling to my attention the hotel/hospitality wellness television phenomenon.

27 Ulrich, "Effects of Health Facility Interior Design on Wellness," 99.
28 Ulrich, "View through a Window May Influence Recovery from Surgery," 420–21.
29 Ulrich, "Effects of Health Facility Interior Design on Wellness," 99.
30 Ibid.
31 Rather than falling into a meaningless relativism, it is more productive to see how particular understandings of TV have accompanied its installation. That is, it is easy to say that, depending on the individual patient and the particular viewing contexts (availability of remote control, individual screen, etc.), television could either be a positive or negative distraction. I could well imagine that *I Love Lucy* could be experienced as painful if the viewing of the program were imposed on, rather than selected by, a viewer. Alternatively, television news could also increase feelings of anxiety or helplessness given the particular context. In this instance, however, I want to foreground the assumptions that have accompanied television's presence in hospitals rather than individualized reception contexts. Though an ethnographic study of hospital television would make a significant contribution to the field, the researcher would need to negotiate patient privacy issues and hospital administration in relation to information gathering.
32 Ulrich, "View through a Window May Influence Recovery from Surgery," 100.
33 For examples of health facilities that have, more recently, recognized the important relationship of design to health and well-being, see Verderber and Fine, *Health Care Architecture in an Era of Radical Transformation*. Of particular significance is their discussion of the design of cancer treatment centers and children's hospitals. Of course, another area that tends to implement supportive design and to recognize the role of architectural space in health and illness is that of hospice architecture.
34 Ulrich, "View through a Window May Influence Recovery from Surgery," 100.
35 For example, several television scholars have addressed the issue of "control" in relation to television viewing; among others: Morley, *The Nationwide Audience*; Allen, *Speaking of Soap Operas*; Ang, *Watching "Dallas"*; Seiter, *Television and New Media Audiences*.
36 Spigel, *Make Room for TV*, 51.
37 McCarthy, *Ambient Television*, 160.
38 Ulrich, "Effects of Health Facility Interior Design on Wellness," 101.
39 Jay W. Collins, "A Combination Television-Radio System for Patients," *Hospitals* 26, no. 11 (1952): 55–56.
40 See Isabelle R. Drumheller, "TV Visiting," *American Journal of Nursing* 59, no. 4 (1959): 522–23; and Lydia Bickford, "Children Visit Patients by Television," *Hospital Management* 82, no. 1 (1956): 51, 62.

41 Stevens, *In Sickness and in Wealth*, 254–55.
42 I am not claiming that private patient rooms were a response to the desegregation of hospitals. I do think, however, that there is a meaningful conjuncture that brings together televisions' installation, the desegregation of hospitals, and the rise in all-private-room hospitals. As *The Modern Hospital* suggested, while patients may not state an overt racial preference, they could do this through code by requesting a private room. See, for example, "Civil Rights Group Challenges Right of Gary Hospital to Ask Patients of Racial Objections," *The Modern Hospital* 101, no. 5 (1963): 174.
43 See, for example, Herbert McLaughlin, "All-Private Room Units: They May Be an Unexpected Bargain," *The Modern Hospital* 110, no. 3 (1968): 100–103. A later article questions the profitability of single-occupancy patient rooms; see "One Patient, One Room: Theory and Practice," *The Modern Hospital* 3, no. 3 (1975): 65. For other discussions of how desegregation and Medicare affected hospitals, see "How Will 'Great Society' Program Affect Hospitals," *The Modern Hospital* 104, no. 1 (1965); and Richard L. Johnson, "Urban Hospitals Face Three Choices: Move, Grow or Change," *The Modern Hospital* 109, no. 5 (1967): 93–96, 160. Several articles from the early 1950s documented responses to the segregation of hospitals. For a variety of perspectives on the issue, see Rev. Jack A. Homer, "Is Segregation Really Necessary?," *The Modern Hospital*, 76, no. 6 (1951): 52–56; C. Rufus Rorem, "No Color Line but No Alternative," *The Modern Hospital* 76, no. 6 (1951): 57–63; and Clyde L. Reynolds, "The Fiscal Results of Segregation," *The Modern Hospital* 76, no. 6 (1951): 64.
44 Lynn Spigel, "Introduction," in Williams, *Television*, xxi.
45 Ibid.
46 Ibid.
47 Ibid.
48 Charles Letourneau, "The Use of Television in Hospitals," *Hospital Management* 97 (May 1964): 52–54.
49 The history of television in hospitals has been documented in a variety of medical journals, most often in terms of medical instruction and the uses of television viewing as a therapeutic tool. See for example, Carpenter, "Psychological Research Using Television"; and Harris, "Television as an Educational Medium in Medicine." Writing about the instructional uses of closed-circuit television in institutional spaces such as primary and secondary schools, Brian Goldfarb has documented the ways educational television was deployed, particularly during the 1960s, as a means of exporting U.S. educational audiovisual materials to other countries. See *Visual Pedagogy*.
50 The question of how to make hospitals less institutional and more homelike in appearance and character, yet modern in terms of technological sophistication, has been a significant concern for administrators, designers, physicians, and staff since the 1920s. This concern is also inflected by contemporary discourses and ideas regarding the nature of health and illness. The

process of humanizing institutions can be understood, in this sense, as a key step in the construction of so-called patient-centered care.
51  See Spigel, *Make Room for TV*, 36–72, 99–135.
52  Meerloo, "Television Addiction and Reactive Apathy."
53  Moore, Chernell, and West, "Television as a Therapeutic Tool," 220.
54  The earliest entry date for television in the *Quarterly Cumulative Index Medicus* is 1953. An entry for 1954 includes a reference to "tele-color clinics." In 1993, telemedicine enters the *Index Medicus* as a new category. For an excellent examination of telemedicine, see Cartwright, "Rural Telemedicine and the Globalization of U.S. Health Care."

### 3: POSITIONING THE PATIENT

1  This is an advertisement from *The Modern Hospital* 75, no. 6 (1950): 129.
2  As Joan Lynaugh and Barbara Brush, historians of hospitals and nursing, describe in *American Nursing*, the effects of post–Second World War developments in science and technology, coupled with an increase in population mobility, growth, and living standards, facilitated a shift in ideas about medical care and accessibility to health care and, specifically, hospital care. Along with these shifts in ideas about medical care, hospitals were expanding on a national level largely due to the proliferation of employer-provided health care and hospitalization insurance. After decades of negotiations and struggles by labor unions, the idea of health care as a basic right began taking hold. Out of the discourses of health care as a productive citizen's basic right, however, the concept of the consumer-patient began to emerge, as hospitals and insurance companies marketed their services to consumers.
3  Spigel explains that one of the concerns about television's entrance into homes in the United States was that it might disrupt familial and gender norms. If television was understood as having the potential to disrupt routine women's work in the home, then it could also replace the father as the new head of the household. Both radio and television broadcasting, cultural critics suggested, could feminize the father and "turn 'real men' into passive homebodies." Television programs such as the "TV or Not TV" premiere episode of *The Honeymooners* depicted men as childlike and feminized by the television, with the wife as caretaker not only of the passive men but of television as well. As Spigel points out, cultural worries over the feminization of the male TV viewer took material form in the turn to do-it-yourself weekend projects for the man of the house, including television manufacturers selling console construction kits. See *Make Room for TV*, 61.
4  Andrews, "Nightingale's Geography," 270–74.
5  Although research on the topic of television and therapeutic discourses is abundant, my use of *therapeutic* and *spatial therapeutics* does not refer to the ways in which television programs represent or engage with a therapeutic ethos. The scholarly literature on the relation between television and

therapeutic discourse, usually but not always, refers to the ways that television programs such as talk shows and some reality programs encourage the physical and mental transformation of participants and viewers through a diagnostic and confessional dynamic. Even in some dramatic programs such as *The Sopranos* (HBO, 1999–2007) or *In Treatment* (HBO, 2008–10), talk therapy is represented as the means toward the transformation (or not) of the characters. Rarely, though, do the accounts of the therapeutic in television programming explain what is meant by this term. Most often references to the therapeutic in analyses of *The Oprah Winfrey Show* (ABC, 1986–2011) or some other programs (the makeover genre of reality television, which I discuss in more detail in the book's conclusion, is particularly rich in terms of a therapeutic ethos) assume that readers know what is meant by this term, and that it has something to do with mental and physical transformation or confessional discourses. Notable exceptions to this assumption include Mimi White's important examination of talk television through Foucault's notion of the confessional, and Eva Illouz's work on public sentimentality and the figure of Oprah Winfrey. When television's therapeutic function is represented in programs, it most often is in the form of a conventional talk-therapy encounter between analyst and client, or between a talk show host and participant, in which the goal is the extraction of truth from the confessing subject. The dynamic is also structured by various types of power formations that tend to position the confessing subject, or the participant who is the receiver of the treatment, on a different level than that of the analyst, therapist, or talk show host. My use of the term *spatial therapeutics* draws on the interdisciplinary work of architects and health and cultural geographers as well as on research representative of what has been called the spatial turn in media studies. See Illouz, *Oprah Winfrey and the Glamour of Misery*; Weber, *Makeover TV*; Shattuc, *The Talking Cure*; and White, *Tele-advising*.

6   Research in the relationship of landscape or the built environment to health spans multiple disciplines, including these texts by cultural geographers, medical/health geographers, medical doctors, architects, and behavioral psychologists: Gesler and Kearns, *Culture/Place/Health*; Gesler, *Cultural Geography of Health Care*; Kellert, Heerwagen, and Mador, eds., *Biophilic Design*; Sternberg, *Healing Spaces*; Williams, ed., *Therapeutic Landscapes*; Andres, "Rethinking the Dynamics between Healthcare and Place"; Gilmour, "Hybrid Space"; Evans, Crooks, and Kingsbury, "Theoretical Injections." Some of these sources are non-U.S. based and include studies of the role of place and structure in health care in countries such as Australia, England, and New Zealand. While the national contexts may be different from the United States, each of these studies emphasizes the importance of natural and built environments in healing and is relevant to my discussion of the role of television and spatial therapeutics in American hospitals.

7   Gesler, "Therapeutic Landscapes," 296.

8   Parr, "Medical Geography."
9   See Evans, Crooks, and Kingsbury, "Theoretical Injections," 718.
10  Ibid. This article uses Foucault and Jacques Lacan to theorize the role of the patient's gaze at the landscape painting and the physician's gaze at the patients within the context of a doctor's office waiting room. The researchers attempt to account for the predominance of landscape paintings in physician waiting rooms and determine how environmental artwork functions in these spaces.
11  C. Victor Twiss, "Interior Decorations in Hospitals," *The Modern Hospital* 7, no. 4 (1916): 337.
12  For other historical documents focusing on the role of interior decorating and design in the management of patient waiting room boredom, see Duane Wanamaker, "How to Select Hospital Furniture," *The Modern Hospital* 17, no. 5 (1921): 433–37; "Does Your Reception Room Attract—or Does It Repel?," *Medical Economics*, September 1927, 36–41; Lucy D. Taylor, "The Problem of the Dark Reception Room," *Medical Economics*, October, 1928, 22–25, 63–65; and Marceille Conkling, "Making the Wait Seem Shorter," *Medical Economics*, June 1929, 12–13, 99–103. A more recent article focusing on the role of interior design is James Falick and James Thomas, "Interesting Interiors Equal Happier Hospitals," *The Modern Hospital* 108, no. 2 (1967): 101–3.
13  Hall, "Encoding/Decoding."
14  Lefebvre, *The Production of Space*, 42.
15  This advertisement is from *Hospital Management*, 70, no. 1 (1950): 11.
16  Foucault elaborates on the history of this relationship in "The Incorporation of the Hospital into Modern Technology." He describes how, among other things, the hospital was transformed from a place where people went to die to a place where people went to be treated for an illness, as well as a site for the "ritual training of the doctor." At the same time that the hospital was becoming medicalized, in Foucault's sense, by "purifying it of its harmful effects," ways of organizing and arranging patients were also changing. Foucault uses the term *medicalize* to stress that the idea of the hospital as a therapeutic instrument is a concept that arose near the end of the eighteenth century. Increasingly, as Foucault observes, the architecture of the hospital became an "agent and instrument of cure in the same category as a dietary regime, bleeding, or other medical actions." The relation of architecture and spatial arrangement to the rise of therapeutic practices was also evident in the organization of patients and the increasingly important site of the patient's bed. The patient's body literally became a source of information about illness, treatment, and prognosis, but it also became a medical record, as "small labels were tied to the wrist," indicating the patient's name, illness, and date of arrival. At the foot of the patient's bed, documents were attached that noted the patient's name and records of doctors' visits, prescribed treat-

ments, and nurses' notes. The patient's body and the patient's bed, in this way, became sites of recordkeeping and information, "formed in the heart of the hospital" and "constituted not only a place of cure but also a place of record and acquisition of knowledge" (151).

17  This advertisement is from *The Modern Hospital* 95, no. 6 (1960): 140.
18  This advertisement is from *The Modern Hospital* 100, no. 3 (1963): 241.
19  This advertisement is from *The Modern Hospital* 105, no. 5 (1965): 208.
20  Earle Howard, "Push-Button Age Hits Hospital," *Today's Health* 36, no. 11 (1958): 10–12.
21  Ibid., 11.
22  This advertisement is from *The Modern Hospital* 105, no. 3 (1968): 123.
23  This advertisement is from *The Modern Hospital* 100, no. 3 (1963): 269.
24  Consumer-patients may in fact not be consoled by television's presence, but rather agitated by it. For one example, television sound coming from an adjacent patient's pillow speaker may be distracting and noisy when the other patient may be trying to sleep, receiving treatment, or having visitors (if it is a semiprivate room). While it is the case that, in recent contexts, consumer-patients may view many different kinds of television content, along with prescription drug commercials, in the hospital, I am more concerned with the assumptions voiced by the advertisements and accompanying trade press that represent the experience of hospital television as spatially therapeutic.

#### 4: TELEVISION IN AND OUT OF THE HOSPITAL

1  Hadacol, a patent medicine with an alcohol content of 12 percent, was advertised during the mid-twentieth century as a vitamin supplement. The Louisiana state senator Dudley J. LeBlanc concocted the tonic; he had no formal medical training but suffered from various aches and pains. Interestingly, LeBlanc at one time hired Hollywood celebrities, including Lucille Ball, Milton Berle, Bob Hope, and others, to promote Hadacol. See Young, *The Medical Messiahs*; and Martin, *Coozan Dudley LeBlanc*. In 1873 Lydia Pinkham created an herbal concoction that she brewed and bottled in her home cellar in Lynn, Massachusetts. She started to market the product as Lydia E. Pinkham's Vegetable Compound for "women's weaknesses." The bottle bore the slogan "Only a Woman Understands Women's Ills." Pinkham, while an early patent medicine maker, has also been referred to as a pioneer in what we now call direct-to-consumer drug advertising. The compound continues to be manufactured and sold today. See Conrad and Leiter, "From Lydia Pinkham to Queen Levitra," 825–38.
2  For an analysis of how pharmaceutical companies advertised psychopharmaceuticals to physicians and later to women (through Prozac), and the gendered features of this marketing history, see Metzl, *Prozac on the Couch*.

Metzl's book provides a history of psychiatry and the rise of pharmacology, as well as an examination of the role that gender played in representing male and female patients from the 1950s to the early 2000s.

3   One way of documenting the economic implications of health care is to consider the rise in medical bankruptcies. Recent data show that the number of bankruptcies attributed to medical problems between 2001 and 2007 rose by 50 percent. For example, from January 1 through June 30, 2007, there were 404,090 bankruptcies filed in the United States. Other data indicate that 62.1 percent of all bankruptcies have a medical basis, and that most cases of medical bankruptcies were filed by middle-class and well-educated consumers who also had health insurance. In addition, the mean age for bankruptcy filing was 44.4, with a monthly mean household income of $2,676 and homes with a market value of $147,776 (for those who owned homes). These data indicate that while the marketing of prescription medications to consumers has increased, when consumer-patients actually become ill (even with health insurance) their capacity to avoid economic hardship depends on their economic assets. In that respect, the medicalization of everyday life, on the one hand, can call attention to medical information that can be useful. On the other hand, our capacity to benefit from the treatments advertised is dependent on a variety of factors, not the least of which is economic capability. This does not necessarily mean that medical marketing messages are resisted, but rather that consumer-patients are still positioned as if they are the ideal subjects of address regardless of whether they can buy the health advertised. For data on medical bankruptcy, see Himmelstein et al., "Medical Bankruptcy in the United States, 2007."

4   Another way that the home is medicalized that has little to do with television, but more to do with the Internet, is through the adoption of telemedicine for home health care. While telemedicine has existed in various forms for almost five decades, new information monitoring and distribution technologies have resituated the individual home as a preferred site for care. I discuss this phenomenon of electronic care (or "e-care"), aging in place, and the 2010 National Broadband Plan in this book's conclusion.

5   Consumer-patients' responses to DTC advertising will be provided in the next chapter. Some surveys indicate that consumer-patients dislike this new mode of advertising, but other research shows that prescription drug advertising is well received by consumer-patients.

6   See Angell, *The Truth about Drug Companies*; DeGrandpre, *The Cult of Pharmacology*; and Petersen, *Our Daily Meds*.

7   Starr, *The Social Transformation of American Medicine*, 79–145.

8   Basara, "Direct-to-Consumer Advertising," 318.

9   Ibid.

10  The first U.S. print prescription drug advertisement directed specifically to consumers appeared in 1981. A Shreveport, Louisiana–based American subsidiary of Boots Pharmaceuticals, a British drug company that also oper-

ates as a retail pharmacy, launched a campaign for Rufen, an ibuprofen product. Also in 1981, Merck Sharp & Dohme released the second print, direct-to-consumer prescription drug advertisement (for Pneumovax, its pneumonia vaccine). The Federal Trade Commission, after the passage in 1962 of the Kefauver-Harris Drug Amendments to the Federal Food, Drug, and Cosmetic Act of 1938, was granted oversight of over-the-counter drug advertising. As an effect of the 1962 Kefauver-Harris Drug Amendments, the FDA was granted regulatory power over prescription drug advertising. At that time, the main concern was the regulation of advertising to physicians and "promotions directed to the medical community," because direct-to-consumer advertising did not yet exist. The actual regulation of drug advertising to physicians and consumers is conducted within the FDA through the Division of Drug Marketing, Advertising, and Communications, under the Center for Drug Evaluation and Research. See the JAMA 112, no. 19 (1939): 1952.

11  Founded in 1847, one of the American Medical Association's main goals was to *professionalize* the role of the physician as *the* medical expert. By the close of the nineteenth century, however, the AMA began to organize against patent medicine sellers and others whom the association considered threats to the professionalization of medicine (including midwives). See Ehrenreich and English, *For Her Own Good*. Before the intervention of the AMA, consuming patent medicines was common, while seeing a physician was a luxury. Nonetheless, the AMA was successful in significantly curtailing the advertising of patent medicines. At issue was the proper dispensing of approved medical advice. In this sense, the congressional passage of the 1906 Pure Food and Drug Act was more than a response to false and fraudulent statements on patent medicine labels; it also limited the popular distribution and circulation of medical information. Because of the decrease in patent medicine advertising to physicians and consumers, drug manufacturers of prescription and patent drugs found alternative means of informing prospective prescribers about their products. One of the ways that patent and prescription drug manufacturers advertised their products was directly to the physician through the practice of detailing.

12  Daniel Carlat, "Dr. Drug Rep," *New York Times Magazine*, November 25, 2007.

13  The relationship between the physician and the detailer has been discussed in professional medical publications such as *JAMA* and the *New England Journal of Medicine*. From critiques of the participatory role of newspapers in relation to nostrum advertising to editorials pointing out the ethical dilemmas presented by drug-company-sponsored university research and lectureships, physicians have at least given editorial attention to this issue from the inside. Apart from resolutions passed by the AMA and physicians' own revisions of behavior, however, the ties between the physician and the pharmaceutical sales representative remain an active arena for the circula-

tion of influence and professional collusion. From a marketing perspective, then, the physician is just as important in the promotion of prescription drugs as is the lay consumer requesting name-brand, non-generic drugs from his or her physician.

14  Apart from resolutions passed by the AMA and various other individual practice–related initiatives, the relation between physicians and pharmaceutical sales methods remains a dirty little secret of medical commerce. This relationship between the physician and pharmaceutical sales representative has also tended to emphasize the ways that the professional is immune to traditional marketing practices.

15  Palumbo and Mullins, "The Development of Direct-to-Consumer Prescription Drug Advertising Regulation," 424.

16  "Drugmakers Reduce Spending on Prescription Drug Advertising," April 16, 2009, http://www.kaiserhealthnews.org/.

17  Gary Gatyas, "IMS Health Reports U.S. Prescription Sales Grew 1.3 Percent in 2008 to $291 Billion," March 19, 2009, http://www.imshelath.com/. IMS Health is a provider of "market intelligence to the pharmaceutical and health care industries."

18  Gilman, *Disease and Representation*, 2.

19  Ibid.

20  Ibid., 3. It is necessary to account, on the one hand, for these representations of consumer-patients that tend to normalize depression and anxiety and, on the other hand, those media representations that stigmatize mental illness—the news media images of Andrea Yates, in particular. Yates, a thirty-nine-year-old wife and mother living in Houston, was found guilty in March 2002 of drowning her five children. Court TV made her private medical records available on its website. Among other medical conditions, Yates was diagnosed and treated (although not consistently) for postpartum depression, psychosis, and schizophrenia. As the drug commercials represent images of normal life made possible through the consumption of a prescription, news images of Andrea Yates, as well as other faces of mental illness, continue to reconstitute the boundaries of a disease-controlled self and a diseased (uncontrolled) other.

21  For an analysis of the distinctions between licit and illicit drugs, see Lenson, *On Drugs*; Jenkins, *Synthetic Panics*; and Plant, *Writing on Drugs*.

22  It should be noted that the push for reform, and the research that went into it, was largely the result of First Lady Hillary Clinton's initiatives rather than President Bill Clinton's work.

23  Lammers and Geist, "The Transformation of Caring in the Light and Shadow of 'Managed Care,'" 49.

24  Paul Noth, *New Yorker*, July 7–14, 2008, 64. See also Gardiner Harris, "As Doctors Write Prescriptions, Drug Companies Write Checks," *New York Times*, June 27, 2004.

25 These are only the utilitarian aspects of drug promotion and selling. The lengths to which drug sales representatives will go to promote their particular products to individual physicians are extraordinary and costly. While my analysis draws on anecdotal information about some of these practices from physicians who have been willing to talk about it (anonymously), rarely, if ever, have these types of professional consumerism been addressed under the rubric of consumer culture studies.

26 Sheryl Gay Stolberg and Jeff Gerth, "High-Tech Stealth Being Used to Sway Doctor Prescriptions," *New York Times*, November 16, 2000.

27 Ibid. As Stolberg and Gerth point out, "only about 40 percent of American doctors are dues-paying members of the AMA," but "the database has detailed personal and professional information, including the D.E.A. number, on all doctors practicing in the United States." Thus the information the AMA sells to pharmaceutical market research firms or to corporations themselves is quite valuable from a marketing perspective.

28 Ibid.

29 For more information regarding the relationship of pharmaceutical sales representatives and physicians, see Andaleeb and Tallman, "Relationships of Physicians with Pharmaceutical Sales Representatives and Pharmaceutical Companies." Andaleeb and Tallman show that while the "physicians see the PSR [pharmaceutical sales representative] as an important source of information, they feel they could get the needed information without the PSR's assistance. . . . They did not view them as a vital part of their practice. Samples and gifts did not seem to be very important to physicians." But the funding provided by continuing medical education did "appear to be important." In other words, "PSRs are yet to be seen by physicians as their partners in delivering better health care at reasonable costs to the ultimate beneficiary, the customer" (87). Given this, it makes sense that pharmaceutical marketers would turn to the customer to attempt to convince him or her of the importance and centrality of the pharmaceutical corporation in their everyday lives.

30 Stolberg and Gerth, "High-Tech Stealth Being Used to Sway Doctor Prescriptions."

31 Bleidt, "Marketing Activities."

32 At the other extreme are consumer-patients who are being taken advantage of by the greedy and manipulative drug industries. Jackie Stacey explains that "patients have traditionally been constructed as passive, compliant and obedient within biomedicine. The expert authority of the medical professional depends upon its exclusivity and its specialization. Medical expertise relies upon keeping a particular domain of knowledge within a specific minority and away from the unenlightened majority." Stacey says "keeping patients 'ignorant' about their illnesses and treatments has long legitimated the wisdom of the medical profession" (*Teratologies*, 205).

33  For information on the television network placement of prescription drug commercials, see Brownfield et al., "Direct-to-Consumer Drug Advertisements on Network Television"; and Frosch et al., "Creating Demand for Prescription Drugs." Regarding physician prescribing behavior, see Kaiser Family Foundation, "Public and Physician Views of Direct-to-Consumer Prescription Drug Advertising," April 2008, http://www.kff.org/; and Kravitz et al., "Influence of Patients' Requests for Direct-to-Consumer Advertised Antidepressants."

34  In 2008 Viagra sponsored the NASCAR driver Mark Martin #6.

35  Text taken from the Public Citizen website, http://citizen.org/.

36  "Twenty of the largest health insurance and drug companies and their trade groups spent nearly $35 million in the first quarter of 2009 [on lobbying], up more than $10 million from the same period in [2008]." For example, Pfizer spent $6.1 million in lobbying, "up 199% from 2008." The Pharmaceutical Research and Manufacturers of America trade group spent $6.9 million, up 91 percent in 2009. See John Fritze, "Lobbying Boosted as Health Care Debate Heats Up," USA Today, June 12, 2009.

37  The keenly perceptive parodies of *Saturday Night Live* are examples of against-the-grain readings of drug commercials. In February 2008, the program presented "Annuale," a parody of a prescription drug commercial in which women take a medication that reduces their menstrual periods to one day per year. The commercial follows the form of a typical drug commercial, with a female voice-over explaining what the drug does, and with different female actors talking about how it has changed their lives (and demonstrating examples of this life-altering behavior). Closing out the commercial is a written list of side effects that scroll over the screen as the voice-over reads the text. One possible side effect includes growing a "leathery tail" and, perhaps, "a second vagina."

38  In the United States the "pharmaceutical industry in 2006 spent $4.8 billion on consumer ads" while the industry "spent $7.2 billion more marketing products to doctors" (Appleby, "Analyzing the Side Effects of Drug Ads"). This data comes from IMS Health, a provider of information for the health care industry. Founded in 1954, its clients include "decision makers in life sciences, payers, providers, or policymakers" (see http://imshealth.com). One of the things that IMS Health tracks is global pharmaceutical sales activity from year to year. Its information appears in a variety of sources from USA Today to publications by the Kaiser Family Foundation.

39  While there are various figures denoting prescription drug advertising expenditures, these were obtained through a medical marketing research firm, IMS Health. Similar figures were reported in *Brandweek*, an advertising and marketing trade journal.

40  Lisa Belkin, "Prime Time Pushers," *Mother Jones*, March/April 2001, 31.

41  This data was generated by the National Institute for Health Care Man-

agement (NIHCM), a lobbying think tank supported largely by health-maintenance organization and insurance-industry executives. NIHCM continues to use data such as these to curb the power of pharmaceutical industries in favor of health-maintenance organizations and the insurance industry.

42   Canon Data Products Group, "DTC Advertising Review and Outlook," special report, PharmaLive.com.

43   While 2005 showed a decrease in direct-to-consumer drug advertising on major television networks, by 2009, spending had increased again. One way to account for the increase in promotional spending in all media, not just television, is that pharmaceutical companies were trying to promote "blockbuster brands" before patent protections expired. See ibid., 1. Cable television networks have seen a rise in pharmaceutical advertising, according to *Broadcasting and Cable*, because of valuable niche markets where Pfizer can advertise Viagra, for example, on ESPN or Spike, and Lipitor on the Food Network. See "Pharmed Out," *Broadcasting and Cable*, September 5, 2005, http://www.broadcastingcable.com/.

44   Kathryn J. Aikin, John L. Swasy, Amie C. Braman, "Patient and Physician Attitudes and Behaviors Associated with DTC Promotion of Prescription Drugs—Summary of FDA Search Results," U.S. Department of Health and Human Services, Food and Drug Administration, Center for Drug Evaluation and Research, November 19, 2004, 5.

45   Ibid., 6–7.

46   Ibid., 6–7.

47   For histories of the managed care medical system, see Stevens, Rosenberg, and Burns, eds., *History and Health Policy in the United States*; and Dranove, *The Economic Evolution of American Health Care*.

48   Indeed, the language of the marketplace was maintained in the debates about health care reform during 2009 and 2010.

### 5: MEDIATED AGENCY

1   That multiple syllable word, the longest in the English language, denotes an actual disease affecting the lungs, caused by inhalation of microscopic silicate or quartz dust.

2   According to the National Association for Home Care and Hospice, in 2004 7.6 million individuals received home-care services from seventeen thousand providers. In 2007 the annual expenditure (including Medicare, Medicaid, and individual spending) for home health care was estimated to be $57.6 billion. See Centers for Medicare and Medicaid Services, Office of the Actuary, "Basic Statistics about Home Care," January 2008, http://www.nahc.org/facts.

3   Loe, *The Rise of Viagra*.
4   The word *pharmaceutical* comes from the Greek word *pharkeutikos*, from *pharmakeus* (preparer of drugs, poisons) and from *pharmakon* (medicine, poison).
5   I thank Ken Nielsen for this comment.
6   See Crawford, "Health as a Meaningful Social Practice."
7   Potts and Tiefer, "Introduction," 267.
8   Watkins, *On the Pill*, 2. See also Marks, *Sexual Chemistry*.
9   Watkins, *On the Pill*, 2.
10  See, for example, Haraway, *Simians, Cyborgs, and Women*; Grosz, *Space, Time and Perversion*; and Balsamo, *Technologies of the Gendered Body*.
11  Tiefer and Potts, "Introduction," 267.
12  Tiefer, "The Viagra Phenomenon," 275.
13  Ibid.
14  Tiefer, "The Viagra Phenomenon," 274.
15  Calasanti and King, "Firming the Floppy Penis," 3.
16  Ibid., 4.
17  Ibid., 5.
18  Where the two categories of masculinity and aging have been most obviously discussed is in relation to health, and particularly the proliferation of feminist critiques of Viagra and other technologies of sexuality. See Moore, *Sperm Counts*.
19  Natasha Singer, "As Doctors Cater to Looks, Skin Patients Wait," *New York Times*, July 28, 2008.
20  Foucault, *Language, Counter-Memory, Practice*, 199–200.
21  See Grace et al., "The Discursive Condition of Viagra."
22  Appearing solid and all-powerful, hegemonic formations (here, white, heterosexual, middle-class, middle-aged men) are actually quite fragile, kind of like the wizard behind the curtain in *The Wizard of Oz* (1939): always devising new and clever ways of maintaining the illusion, and the effect, of power.
23  The naming of drugs, as with the branding of other commodities, is a complex process designed to denote as well as connote. Think of the various disorders and conditions and the brand names for each of the following categories:

Allergies: Allegra (Sanofi-Aventis), Clarinex (Schering-Plough), Claritin (Schering-Plough), Flonase (GlaxoSmithKline), Nasonex (Schering-Plough), Zyrtec (McNeil-PPC)

Depression: Celexa (Forest), Effexor (Wyeth), Paxil (GlaxoSmithKline), Prozac (Eli Lilly), Remeron (Organon), Wellbutrin (GlaxoSmithKline), Zoloft (Pfizer)

Sleep Disorder: Ambien (Sanofi-Aventis), Lunesta (Sunovion), Rozerem (Takeda), Sonata (King)

Each brand name connects through vowel and consonant aural combinations or through evocative connotations in which the name reminds the consumer of another word—such as "Paxil" and "peace," or "Effexor" and "effective," both prescription drugs for depression; or "Flonase" and "flow," when nasal allergies attack.

24 Loe, *The Rise of Viagra*, 53.
25 Halberstam, *Female Masculinity*, 234.
26 Ibid., 2.
27 Kristin Davis, "Marketers, Take Note: Baby Boomers Have Lots of Money to Spend," *U.S. News and World Report*, March 14, 2005, http://www.agewave.com/.
28 Jeff MacGregor, "The New Electoral Sex Symbol: NASCAR Dad," *New York Times*, January 18, 2004.
29 Michael Johnsen, "Convenience Is a Key Driver for These Old-School Shoppers," *Drug Store News*, June 21, 2004, http://www.accessmylibrary.com/.
30 While it is possible that all texts—from mass media products such as film, television programs, advertising in all its shapes and incarnations, and music, to fashion and art—are intertextual to the extent that meaning making occurs only *in relation* to certain kinds of awareness of other texts and experiences, it is not the case that all texts are parodic or that they display what Jonathan Gray has called "critical intertextuality." See Gray, *Watching with "The Simpsons."*
31 Kelly Simmons quoted in Stuart Elliott, "Viagra, with a Wink and a Nudge, Joins Its Racier Rivals on Their Turf," *New York Times*, August 17, 2004.
32 Stuart Elliott, "Viagra and the Battle of the Awkward Ads," *New York Times*, April 25, 2004. Unfortunately, Carlin was not able to realize this potential addition to his insightful comedy, as he died in June 2008.
33 Loe, *The Rise of Viagra*, 59.
34 In contrast to the serious or romantic early ads, featuring the dancing couples and the former senator and 1996 Republican presidential candidate Bob Dole, more recent Viagra ads show a sense of playfulness that can be read, on one level, as an indicator of the comfort that Viagra enjoys as the best-selling erectile dysfunction prescription drug.
35 Theresa Howard, "Viagra Ads Try to Inform without Embarrassing," *USA Today*, August 24, 2003.
36 Baglia, *The Viagra AdVenture*, 78. With the disclosure of steroid use among Major League Baseball players (Palmeiro included), this further complicates the idea of the natural male body as simulated and stimulated through artificial means—an equally rich example of the reclamation of strength and performative vitality and value (in terms of player's contracts) of the aging male.
37 Melody Petersen, "A New Rival to Viagra Enlists the N.F.L. to Put a Masculine Face on a Sensitive Subject," *New York Times*, July 18, 2003.
38 Ibid.

39  Melody Petersen, "Pfizer, Facing Competition from Other Drug Makers, Looks for a Younger Market for Viagra," *New York Times*, February 13, 2002.
40  Vares and Braun, "Spreading the Word, but What Word Is That?," 317.
41  Elizabeth Cohen, "Five Symptoms Men Shouldn't Ignore," CNN.com, July 12, 2008.
42  McAlexander, Schouten, and Koenig, "Building Brand Community," 38.
43  Jackson, *Winning and Keeping Industrial Customers*, xi (emphasis added).
44  The AIDS Health Care Foundation criticized Viagra's Viva Viagra campaign for promoting irresponsible sexual practices through the Las Vegas reference. Moreover, although Pfizer's advertisements emphasize heterosexual monogamous sex, their website does have a partner section. Gay men and men who have sex with men also use Viagra, but these users seem to be primarily studied for their recreational use of the drug rather than their actual need. For example, the medical journal *Sexually Transmitted Infections* published a study conducted in 2004 about the recreational use of Viagra among men who have sex with men. The researchers found that "recreational use of Viagra was relatively common among men, regardless of age or HIV serostatus. Viagra was associated with men's substance abuse behaviour rather than their sexual risk behaviour." Crosby and DiClemente, "Use of Recreational Viagra among Men Having Sex with Men," 466.
45  By 2010 highly popular primetime broadcast dramas such as *24*, *Lost*, and *Heroes* incorporated into their storylines various languages other than English and began to use subtitles. In some ways, one can understand this as an acknowledgment of a diverse and narrowcast audience, but also as a means of increasing brand loyalty for television networks and products across an ethnically and racially diverse demographic field.
46  Near the end of the song and commercial, a male voice-over begins to give viewers instructions and information about Viagra: "Talk to your doctor about Viagra, America's most prescribed treatment for erectile dysfunction. Learn more at Viagra.com. Ask your doctor if your heart is healthy enough for sex. Don't take Viagra if you take nitrates for chest pain, as it may cause an unsafe drop in blood pressure. Side effects may include headache, flushing, upset stomach, and abnormal vision. To avoid long-term injuries, stop taking Viagra and call your doctor right away if you experience a sudden decrease in vision or an erection lasting longer than four hours." The warning highlights the fact that, if any consumer-patient has any of these conditions, Viagra can actually do more harm than good. Rather than facilitating sexual health, Viagra can cause or exacerbate many other medical problems.
47  "Got me a honey . . . / Now this lonesome toad is / Sick of the road / I can't wait (I can't wait) / I can't wait to go home / Viva Viagra! / Viva! Viva! Viagra!"
48  In a series of fortuitous events, Lucky gets back his engine and wins the race, as well as the girl, Rusty Martin (Ann-Margret), a Flamingo Hotel swimming

instructor, pool manager, and dancer who can match Lucky's moves with her own. The film includes some famous songs, such as Elvis's version of Ray Charles's "What'd I Say" and a duet with Ann-Margret, "The Lady Loves Me" (as well as the theme song, of course, "Viva Las Vegas").

49 "Bright light city gonna set my soul / Gonna set my soul on fire / Got a whole lot of money that's ready to burn . . . / Viva Las Vegas, Viva Las Vegas!" (words and music by Doc Pomus and Mort Shuman).

50 That the commercial references Presley also demonstrates a certain nostalgic vision for a historical moment in the construction of male sexuality *before* Viagra, the Playboy moment, in which, according to this logic, sex was simply sex, without the need for sexuopharmaceutical intervention.

51 Singing about the merits of Viagra did not originate with the "Viva Viagra" campaign, but was actually demonstrated in two earlier intertextual commercials: one commercial that uses "Good Mornin'" from *Singin' in the Rain* (Stanley Donen, 1952) and "We Are the Champions" by Queen. Pfizer's "We Are the Champions" commercial appeared on American broadcast television in 2004, but it was developed by a Canadian advertising agency, Taxi, and was first shown on Canadian television. The commercial begins with a crane shot of an obviously artificial suburban street, and then the camera cuts to a medium shot of a white, middle-aged man leaping out of his front door. Extending his arms as Freddie Mercury begins to sing "We Are the Champions," the man leaps and dances through a white picket fence to the sidewalk and street, where he greets other men who are also leaping and dancing. A mail carrier throws his letters and parcels in the air, a businessman empties his briefcase of documents, and an older woman waters her plants as she watches in amazement. Then, men—including one in a wheelchair—and women all gather in the street as Freddie Mercury reaches the refrain of the song. The commercial ends with a big blue pill labeled "Viagra" in the center of the screen with the words "Talk to your doctor" underneath.

The commercial gushes with fun and pleasure, emphasizing an approach to male sexuality that is playful and humorous. This commercial, which was edited for broadcast in the United States (originally, in a risqué visual pun, a man was watering his yard, but that was changed to a woman with a hose), conveys a playful sense of male sexuality, one in which men and woman are shown together, by themselves, and men are shown celebrating with other men.

52 This particular campaign, on television and the website, ended in 2009, but a new campaign has taken its place. My analysis is based on the 2007–9 campaign. Viagra's promotion in 2010 downplays the folksy and humorous perspective for a more serious approach. The webpages that I describe here are no longer active, but Viagra still maintains a significant web presence as well as advertisements on television, in magazines, and through its sponsorship of NASCAR.

53 The term *habitus* comes from Bourdieu's *Distinction*, 6. In his use of the term, Bourdieu designated fields within which particular classes recognized themselves and identified others based on a sense of shared taste. For Bourdieu, taste involves "systems of dispositions (habitus) characteristic of the different classes and class fractions. Taste classifies the classifier." Pfizer constructs a series of dispositions that are based on class, but which are also based on commonsense notions of what it means to be a sexually healthy male citizen.

54 White, *The Body and the Screen*, 1.

55 The value card was apparently discontinued as of 2010. Gone are the links for value cards, and in their place are links for information presented in a doctor's office mise en scène. The analysis of the earlier campaign serves as a historical snapshot of a particular moment in the ongoing marketing of Viagra. The 2011 Viagra website declares that "This Is the Age of Taking Action" and features a series of men, some dressed as physicians in white lab coats, others working on small aircraft or automobile engines, and other men, who are casually dressed, looking directly at the viewer to encourage identification. The website in 2011 also offers an interesting warning to be wary of Viagra counterfeiters.

56 Crawshaw, "Governing the Healthy Male Citizen," 1607.

57 Weber, *Makeover TV*, 39.

58 The U.S. Census categorizes middle age as ranging from thirty-five to fifty-four. Over sixty-four years of age is considered old. These categories, based only on years lived, do not, of course, take into account other cultural and social features of what it means to age, and they certainly vary from individual to individual as to how each person feels being a particular age. Youth and old age are, to a degree, also cultural categories constructed on assumptions about age, gender, sexuality, class, and race. For example, one cultural connotation of being an old man is that this means one is wise, while another cultural connotation suggests limitation, inaction, immobility, and fragility.

59 For a detailed discussion of the history of male vital power from the ancient Greeks to contemporary cultures, see McLaren, *Impotence*. Among the historical features of impotence discussed by McLaren is the story of how Magnus Hirschfeld's Institute for Sexual Science in Germany funded its work through the sale of "Testifortan," a pharmaceutical for the treatment of impotence, to medical professionals. McLaren notes that, "after 1929, it was sold to the general public as Titus Pearls," and is mentioned in, among other texts, Alfred Doblin's novel *Alexanderplatz* (1931), "in which the hero is subjected to advertisements for Testifortan" (194).

60 Burri and Dumit, eds., "Introduction," *Biomedicine as Culture*, 4.

61 Ibid.

## CONCLUSION

1. "Oprah Winfrey and Discovery Communications to Form New Joint Venture," press release, Discovery Communications, January 15, 2008, http://corporate.discovery.com/.
2. Harpo and Discovery will share ownership of the new network, with each company owning 50 percent. But Winfrey will have total control of content and programming decisions. See Marisa Guthrie and Anne Becker, "Oprah, Discovery Team up on New Network," *Broadcasting and Cable* 138, no. 3 (2008): 27.
3. For Discovery Health's parent company, Discovery Communications, the deal rebrands one of many outlets controlled by an entity that touts itself on its website as the "number one nonfiction media company reaching more than 1.5 billion subscribers in over 170 countries. Discovery's 100-plus worldwide networks are led by Discovery Channel, TLC, Animal Planet, The Science Channel, Discovery Health and HD Theater, with digital media properties including HowStuffWorks.com."
4. As indicated in the 2008 Beta Research Brand Identity of Basic Cable/Broadcast Networks Study, for the past eight years viewers have ranked Discovery Channel highest among cable networks. See "Discovery Channel Ranks as the Highest-Quality Network," April 29, 2008, http://corporate.discovery.com/.
5. Banet-Weiser, "The Nickelodeon Brand," 234.
6. "Oprah Winfrey and Discovery Communications to Form New Joint Venture."
7. Ibid.
8. "Robin Schwartz Named President of OWN," June 18, 2008, http://corporate.discovery.com/.
9. Debbi K. Swanson, "Cable's Media Front a Mixed Bag," *Advertising Age* 72, no. 16 (2001): S24.
10. Ibid.
11. PR Newswire Association, "Discovery Communications Announces Merck Marketing Executive Leonard J. Tacconi as New President of Discovery Health Media," PRNewswire.com, September 6, 2006.
12. Weber, *Makeover TV*, 259.
13. Dyer, *Only Entertainment*, 17.
14. See, for example, Ouellette and Hay, *Better Living through Reality TV*; McMurria, "Desperate Citizens and Good Samaritans"; McCarthy, "Reality Television"; Heller, *Makeover Television*.
15. McCarthy, "Reality Television," 19.
16. A medical study published in 2007 in *Plastic and Reconstructive Surgery* indicates that reality television makeover programs that feature cosmetic plastic surgery have an influence on patients' decisions to such procedures. Of forty-two patients, 57 percent "reported a greater influence from tele-

vision and the media to pursue cosmetic plastic surgery," and "felt more knowledgeable about plastic surgery in general and believed that plastic surgery reality TV shows were more similar to real life than low-intensity viewers did. In addition, four out of five people reported television directly influenced them to pursue a cosmetic plastic surgery procedure." Programs included in the study were *Extreme Makeover* (ABC), *The Swan* (Fox), *I Want a Famous Face* (MTV), *Plastic Surgery: Before and After* (TLC), *Dr. 90210* (E!), and *Miami Slice* (Bravo). See Crockett, Pruzinsky, and Persing, "The Influence of Plastic Surgery Reality TV on Cosmetic Surgery Patient Expectations and Decision Making," 316.

17 Self-transformation reality shows such as *The Biggest Loser* are more than mere tools for humiliation. For viewers who do not have familial or social support systems from which they may be able to draw for weight-loss inspiration and encouragement, weight-loss programs may function as empowering and instructive televisual community. For those viewers who cannot afford the luxury of a personal trainer but who want to learn how to use resistance training to tone muscle, programs such as Bravo's *Work Out* might be a means to this end.

18 McCarthy, "Reality Television," 19.

19 My optimistic disposition points me in the direction of ways that indicate how health can be a national priority. One has to look no further than the 2010 passage of health care reform to see that, at least to a certain degree, the state recognizes the links between citizenship and health, or citizenship and "insurance care." And there are initiatives such as First Lady Michelle Obama's "Let's Move" national campaign against childhood obesity. While not official state programs, "Let's Move" and Mrs. Obama's high-profile installation of a vegetable garden on the White House lawn emphasize an individual as well as institutional involvement in health care advocacy.

20 The debate on obesity and health continues with the publication of a study in the *Archives of Internal Medicine*. While it is represented as commonsensical in weight-loss shows that smaller-sized people are healthier by virtue of not being overweight (relative to normative body proportions), medical experts are not so sure: "Among U.S. adults, there is a high prevalence of clustering of cardiometabolic abnormalities among normal-weight individuals and a high prevalence of overweight and obese individuals who are metabolically healthy. Further study into the physiologic mechanisms underlying these different phenotypes and their impact on health is needed." Wildman et al., "The Obese without Cardiometabolic Risk Factor Clustering and the Normal Weight with Cardiometabolic Risk Factor Clustering," 1617.

21 Andrew Adam Newman, "No Actors, Just Patients in Unvarnished Spots for Hospitals," *New York Times*, May 26, 2009.

22 Ibid.

23 Pam Belluck, "Webcast Your Brain Surgery? Hospitals See Marketing Tool," *New York Times*, May 25, 2009.
24 Ryan Singel, "FCC to Release Ambitious, but Pragmatic, National Broadband Plan," March 15, 2010, http://www.wired.com/.
25 "Broadband Action Agenda," National Broadband Plan, http://www.broadband.gov/plan/broadband-action-agenda.html.
26 A video recording of this hearing, "Aging in Place: The National Broadband Plan and Bringing Health Care Technology Home," is available on the U.S. Senate's Special Committee on Aging website: http://aging.senate.gov/hearing_detail.cfm?id=324102&.

## Selected Bibliography

Acland, Charles. "Take Two: Post-Fordist Discourses of the Corporate and the Corporeal." In *When Pain Strikes*, edited by Bill Burns, Cathy Busby, and Kim Sawchuk, 195–212. Minneapolis: University of Minnesota Press, 1999.

Adams, Annmarie. *Medicine by Design: The Architect and the Modern Hospital, 1893–1943*. Minneapolis: University of Minnesota Press, 2008.

Allen, Robert C. *Speaking of Soap Operas*. Chapel Hill: University of North Carolina Press, 1985.

Allen, Robert C., and Douglas Gomery. *Film History: Theory and Practice*. New York: McGraw-Hill, 1993.

Andaleeb, Syed Saad, and Robert F. Tallman. "Relationships of Physicians with Pharmaceutical Sales Representatives and Pharmaceutical Companies: An Exploratory Study." *Health Marketing Quarterly* 13, no. 4 (1996): 79–89.

Andres, Gavin J. "Rethinking the Dynamics between Healthcare and Place: Therapeutic Geographies in Treatment and Care Practices." *Area* 36, no. 3 (2004): 307–18.

Andrews, G. J. "Nightingale's Geography." *Nursing Inquiry* 10, no. 4 (2003): 270–74.

Ang, Ien. *Watching "Dallas": Soap Opera and the Melodramatic Imagination*. London: Methuen, 1985.

Angell, Marcia. *The Truth about Drug Companies: How They Deceive Us and What to Do about It*. Random House: New York, 2004.

Appleby, Julie. "Analyzing the Side Effects of Drug Ads." *USA Today*, February 29, 2008.

Atkin, Charles, and Lawrence Wallack, eds. *Communication and Public Health: Complexities and Conflicts*. Thousand Oaks, Calif.: Sage, 1990.

Baglia, Jay. *The Viagra AdVenture: Masculinity, Media and the Performance of Sexual Health.* New York: Peter Lang, 2005.

Balsamo, Ann. *Technologies of the Gendered Body: Reading Cyborg Women.* Durham: Duke University Press, 1995.

Banet-Weiser, Sarah. "The Nickelodeon Brand: Buying and Selling the Audience." In *Cable Visions: Television beyond Broadcasting,* edited by Sarah Banet-Weiser, Cynthia Chris, and Anthony Freitas, 234–52. New York: New York University Press, 2007.

Basara, Lisa Ruby. "Direct-to-Consumer Advertising: Today's Issues and Tomorrow's Outlook." *Journal of Drug Issues* 22, no. 2 (1992): 317–30.

Berger, Maurice, Brian Wallis, and Simon Watson, eds. *Constructing Masculinity.* London: Routledge, 1995.

Bleidt, Barry. "Marketing Activities: The Keystone of Capitalism—Increasing the Availability of Prescription Drugs through Pharmaceutical Promotion." *Journal of Drug Issues* 22, no. 2 (1992): 277–93.

Bourdieu, Pierre. *Distinction: A Social Critique of the Judgment of Taste.* Translated by Richard Nice. London: Routledge, 1984.

Braun, Marta. *Picturing Time: The Work of Etienne Jules-Marey.* Chicago: University of Chicago Press, 1995.

Brock, Pope. *Charlatan: America's Most Dangerous Huckster, the Man Who Pursued Him, and the Age of Flimflam.* New York: Crown, 2008.

Brownfield, E. D., J. M. Bernhardt, J. L. Phan, M. V. Williams, and R. M. Parker. "Direct-to-Consumer Drug Advertisements on Network Television: An Exploration of Quantity, Frequency, and Placement." *Journal of Health Communication* 9, no. 6 (2004): 491–97.

Burri, Regula Valerie, and Joseph Dumit, eds. *Biomedicine as Culture: Instrumental Practices, Technoscientific Knowledge, and New Modes of Life.* New York: Routledge, 2007.

Calasanti, Toni, and Neal King. "Firming the Floppy Penis." *Men and Masculinities* 8, no. 1 (2005): 3–23.

Carpenter, C. R. "Psychological Research Using Television." *American Psychologist* 10, no. 10 (1955): 606–10.

Cartwright, Lisa. "Rural Telemedicine and the Globalization of U.S. Health Care." In *Biotechnology and Culture: Bodies, Anxieties, Ethics,* edited by Paul Brodwin, 241–63. Bloomington: Indiana University Press, 2001.

———. *Screening the Body: Tracing Medicine's Visual Culture.* Minneapolis: University of Minnesota Press, 1995.

Clarke, Adele, Jennifer Fishman, Jennifer Fosket, Laura Mamo, and Janet Shim. "Biomedicalization: Technoscientific Transformations of Health, Illness, and U.S. Biomedicine." *American Sociological Review* 68, no. 2 (2003): 161–94.

Conrad, Peter, and Valerie Leiter, "From Lydia Pinkham to Queen Levitra: Direct-to-Consumer Advertising and Medicalization." *Sociology of Health and Illness* 30, no. 6 (2008): 825–38.

Couldry, Nick, and Anna McCarthy, eds. *MediaSpace: Place, Scale, and Culture in a Media Age.* New York: Routledge, 2004.

Crawford, Robert. "Health as a Meaningful Social Practice." *Health: An Interdisciplinary Journal for the Social Study of Health, Illness and Medicine* 10, no. 4 (2006): 401–20.

Crawshaw, Paul. "Governing the Healthy Male Citizen: Men, Masculinity and Popular Health in *Men's Health* Magazine." *Social Science and Medicine* 65, no. 8 (2007): 1606–18.

Crimp, Douglas, ed. AIDS: *Cultural Analysis/Cultural Activism.* Cambridge: MIT Press, 1988.

Crockett, Richard J., Thomas Pruzinsky, and John A. Persing. "The Influence of Plastic Surgery Reality TV on Cosmetic Surgery Patient Expectations and Decision Making." *Plastic and Reconstructive Surgery* 120, no. 1 (2007): 316–24.

Crosby, R., and R. J. DiClemente. "Use of Recreational Viagra among Men Having Sex with Men." *Sexually Transmitted Infections* 80, no. 6 (2004): 466–68.

DeCordova, Richard. *Picture Personalities: The Emergence of the Star System in America.* Champaign: University of Illinois Press, 1990.

DeGrandpre, Richard. *The Cult of Pharmacology: How America Became the World's Most Troubled Drug Culture.* Durham: Duke University Press, 2006.

Douglas, Susan. *Listening In: Radio and the American Imagination.* New York: Times Books, 1999.

Dranove, David. *The Economic Evolution of American Health Care: From Marcus Welby to Managed Care.* Baltimore: Johns Hopkins University Press, 2000.

Draper, Ellen. "Controversy Has Probably Destroyed Forever the Context: *The Miracle* and Movie Censorship in America in the 1950s." In *Controlling Hollywood: Censorship and Regulation in the Studio Era,* edited by Matthew Bernstein, 186–205. New Brunswick: Rutgers University Press, 1999.

Dumit, Joseph. *Picturing Personhood: Brain Scans and Biomedical Identity.* Princeton: Princeton University Press, 2003.

Dyer, Richard. *Only Entertainment.* London: Routledge, 1992.

Ehrenreich, Barbara, and Deirdre English. *For Her Own Good: Two Centuries of Experts' Advice to Women.* New York: Anchor, 1978.

Erni, John. *Unstable Frontiers: Technomedicine and the Cultural Politics of "Curing" AIDS.* Minneapolis: University of Minnesota Press, 1994.

Evans, Joshua D., Valorie A. Crooks, and Paul T. Kingsbury. "Theoretical Injections: On the Therapeutic Aesthetics of Medical Spaces." *Social Science and Medicine* 69 (2009): 716–21.

Foucault, Michel. *The Care of the Self: The History of Sexuality, Volume 3.* New York: Random House, 1986.

———. "The Incorporation of the Hospital into Modern Technology." In *Space, Knowledge and Power: Foucault and Geography,* edited by Jeremy Crampton and Stuart Elden, 141–52. Aldershot: Ashgate, 2007.

———. *Language, Counter-Memory, Practice: Selected Essays and Interviews by Michel Foucault*. Edited by Donald F Bouchard. Ithaca: Cornell University Press, 1988.

Friedman, Lester. "Introduction: Through the Looking Glass: Medical Culture and the Media." In *Cultural Sutures: Medicine and Media*, edited by Lester Friedman, 1–11. Durham: Duke University Press, 2004.

Frosch, Dominick L., Patrick M. Krueger, Robert C. Hornik, Peter F. Cronholm, and Frances K. Barg. "Creating Demand for Prescription Drugs: A Content Analysis of Television Direct-to-Consumer Advertising." *Annals of Family Medicine* 5, no. 6 (2007): 6–13.

Gamson, Joshua. *Freaks Talk Back: Tabloid Talk Shows and Sexual Nonconformity*. Chicago: University of Chicago Press, 1999.

Gesler, Wilbert. *Cultural Geography of Health Care*. Pittsburgh: University of Pittsburgh Press, 1991.

———. "Therapeutic Landscapes: An Evolving Theme." *Health and Place* 11, no. 4 (2005): 295–97.

Gesler, Wilbert, and Robin Kearns. *Culture/Place/Health*. New York: Routledge, 2001.

Gilman, Sander. *Disease and Representation: Images of Illness from Madness to AIDS*. Ithaca: Cornell University Press, 1988.

———. *Picturing Health and Illness: Images of Identity and Difference*. Baltimore: Johns Hopkins University Press, 1995.

Gilmour, Jean. "Hybrid Space: Constituting the Hospital as a Home Space for Patients." *Nursing Inquiry* 13, no. 1 (2006): 16–22.

Goldfarb, Brian. *Visual Pedagogy: Media Culture in and beyond the Classroom*. Durham: Duke University Press, 2002.

Gomery, Douglas. *Shared Pleasures: A History of Movie Presentation in the United States*. Madison: University of Wisconsin Press, 1992.

Grace, Victoria, Annie Potts, Nicola Gavey, and Tiina Vares. "The Discursive Condition of Viagra." *Sexualities* 9, no. 3 (2006): 295–314.

Gray, Jonathan. *Watching with "The Simpsons": Television, Parody, and Intertextuality*. London: Routledge, 2006.

Grossberg, Lawrence. "The In-Difference of Television." *Screen* 28, no. 2 (1987): 34–35.

Grosz, Elizabeth. *Space, Time and Perversion: Essays on the Politics of Bodies*. New York: Routledge, 1995.

Gunning, Tom. "In Your Face: Physiognomy, Photography, and the Gnostic Mission of Early Film." *Modernism/Modernity* 4, no. 1 (1997): 1–29.

Halberstam, Judith. *Female Masculinity*. Durham: Duke University Press, 1998.

Hall, Stuart. "Encoding/Decoding." In *Culture, Media, Language: Working Papers in Cultural Studies, 1972–79*, edited by Stuart Hall, Dorothy Hobson, Andrew Lowe, and Paul Willis, 128–38. London: Hutchinson, 1980.

Haraway, Donna. *Simians, Cyborgs, and Women: The Reinvention of Nature*. New York: Routledge, 1991.

Harris, Jerome J. "Television as an Educational Medium in Medicine: An Historical Purview." *Journal of Medical Education* 41, no. 1 (1966): 1–19.
Heller, Dana. *Makeover Television: Realities Remodeled.* London: I. B. Tauris, 2007.
Hilmes, Michele. *Radio Voices: American Broadcasting, 1922–1952.* Minneapolis: University of Minnesota Press, 1997.
Himmelstein, David U., Deborah Thorne, Elizabeth Warren, and Steffie Woolhandler. "Medical Bankruptcy in the United States, 2007: Results of a National Study." *American Journal of Medicine* 20, no. 10 (2009): 1–6.
Illouz, Eva. *Oprah Winfrey and the Glamour of Misery: An Essay on Popular Culture.* New York: Columbia University Press, 2003.
Jackson, Barbara Bund. *Winning and Keeping Industrial Customers.* Lexington, Mass.: Lexington Books, 1985.
Jackson, Lorraine D., and Bernard K. Duffy. *Health Communication Research: A Guide to Developments and Directions.* Westport, Conn.: Greenwood Press, 1998.
Jenkins, Phillip. *Synthetic Panics: The Symbolic Politics of Designer Drugs.* New York: New York University Press, 1999.
Jowett, Garth S. "A Capacity for Evil: The 1915 Supreme Court *Mutual* Decision." In *Controlling Hollywood: Censorship and Regulation in the Studio Era*, edited by Matthew Bernstein, 16–40. New Brunswick: Rutgers University Press, 1999.
Kellert, Stephen, Judith Heerwagen, and Martin Mador, eds. *Biophilic Design: The Theory, Science and Practice of Bringing a Building to Life.* Hoboken: Wiley, 2008.
Kraut, Alan M. *Silent Travelers: Germs, Genes, and the "Immigrant Menace."* Baltimore: Johns Hopkins University Press, 1995.
Kravitz, R. L., R. M. Epstein, M. D. Feldman, C. E. Franz, R. Azari, M. S. Wilkes, L. Hinton, and P. Franks. "Influence of Patients' Requests for Direct-to-Consumer Advertised Antidepressants: A Randomized Controlled Trial." *JAMA* 293, no. 16 (2005): 1995–2002.
Lammers, John C., and Patricia Geist. "The Transformation of Caring in the Light and Shadow of 'Managed Care.'" *Health Communication* 9, no. 1 (1997): 45–60.
Leavitt, Judith Walzer. *Typhoid Mary: Captive to the Public's Health.* New York: Putnam, 1996.
Lee, R. Alton. *The Bizarre Careers of John R. Brinkley.* Lexington: University Press of Kentucky, 2002.
Lefebvre, Henri. *The Production of Space.* Translated by Donald Nicholson-Smith. Oxford: Blackwell, 1991.
Lenson, David. *On Drugs.* Minneapolis: University of Minnesota Press, 1995.
Loe, Meika. *The Rise of Viagra: How the Little Blue Pill Changed Sex in America.* New York: New York University Press, 2004.

Lynaugh, Joan E., and Barbara L. Brush. *American Nursing: From Hospitals to Health Systems*. Cambridge: Blackwell, 1996.

Marks, Lara V. *Sexual Chemistry: A History of the Contraceptive Pill*. New Haven: Yale University Press, 2001.

Martin, Floyd Clay. *Coozan Dudley LeBlanc: From Huey Long to Hadacol*. Gretna, La.: Pelican, 1973.

McAlexander, James H., John W. Schouten, and Harold F. Koenig. "Building Brand Community." *Journal of Marketing* 66, no. 1 (2002): 38–54.

McCarthy, Anna. *Ambient Television: Visual Culture and Public Space*. Durham: Duke University Press, 2001.

———. "Reality Television: A Neoliberal Theater of Suffering." *Social Text* 93, no. 4 (2007): 17–41.

McLaren, Angus. *Impotence: A Cultural History*. Chicago: University of Chicago Press, 2007.

McMurria, John. "Desperate Citizens and Good Samaritans: Neoliberalism and Makeover Reality TV." *Television and New Media* 9, no. 4 (2008): 305–32.

Meerloo, Joost A. M. "Television Addiction and Reactive Apathy." *Journal of Nervous and Mental Disorders* 120 (1954): 290.

Metzl, Jonathan Michel. *Prozac on the Couch: Prescribing Gender in the Era of Wonder Drugs*. Durham: Duke University Press, 2003.

Moore, F. J., E. Chernell, and J. J. West. "Television as a Therapeutic Tool." *Archives of General Psychiatry* 12, no. 27 (1965): 217–21.

Moore, Lisa Jean. *Sperm Counts: Overcome by Man's Most Precious Fluid*. New York: New York University Press, 2008.

Moran, James M. *There's No Place Like Home Video*. Minneapolis: University of Minnesota Press, 2002.

Morley, David. *The Nationwide Audience: Structure and Decoding*. London: British Film Institute, 1980.

Musser, Charles. *High-Class Moving Pictures*. Princeton: Princeton University Press, 1991.

Ostherr, Kirsten. *Cinematic Prophylaxis: Globalization and Contagion in the Discourse of World Health*. Durham: Duke University Press, 2005.

Ouellette, Laurie, and James Hay. *Better Living through Reality TV: Television and Post-welfare Citizenship*. Hoboken: Wiley-Blackwell, 2008.

Palumbo, Francis B., and Daniel C. Mullins. "The Development of Direct-to-Consumer Prescription Drug Advertising Regulation." *Food and Drug Law Journal* 57, no. 3 (2002): 423–43.

Parr, Hester. "Medical Geography: Care and Caring." *Progress in Human Geography* 27, no. 2 (2003): 212–21.

Patton, Cindy. *Inventing AIDS*. London: Routledge, 1990.

Paul, Terry. "Relationship Marketing for Health Care Providers." *Journal of Health Care Marketing* 8, no. 3 (1988): 20–25.

Peiss, Kathy. *Cheap Amusements: Working Women and Leisure in Turn-of-the Century Chicago*. New Brunswick: Rutgers University Press, 1998.

Peters, Thomas J., and Robert H. Waterman. *In Search of Excellence: Lessons from America's Best-Run Companies*. New York: Collins Business, 2001.

Petersen, Melody. *Our Daily Meds: How the Pharmaceutical Companies Transformed Themselves into Slick Marketing Machines and Hooked the Nation on Prescription Drugs*. New York: Farrar, Straus and Giroux, 2008.

Plant, Sadie. *Writing on Drugs*. New York: Picador, 1999.

Porter, Roy. *Madness: A Brief History*. New York: Oxford University Press, 2003.

Potts, Annie. "'The Essence of the Hard-On': Hegemonic Masculinity and the Cultural Construction of 'Erectile Dysfunction.'" *Men and Masculinities* 3, no. 1 (2000): 85–103.

Potts, Annie, and Leonore Tiefer. "Introduction." *Sexualities* 9, no. 3 (2006): 267–72.

Price, Janet, and Margrit Shildrick, eds. *Vital Signs: Feminist Reconfigurations of the Bio/logical Body*. Edinburgh: Edinburgh University Press, 1998.

Reagan, Leslie J., Nancy Tomes, and Paula A. Treichler, eds. *Medicine's Moving Pictures: Medicine, Health, and Bodies in American Film and Television*. Rochester: University of Rochester Press, 2008.

Reid, T. R. *The Healing of America: A Global Quest for Better, Cheaper, and Fairer Health Care*. New York: Penguin, 2009.

Riggs, Karen. *Mature Audiences: Television in the Lives of Elders*. New Brunswick: Rutgers University Press, 1998.

Risse, Guenter B. *Mending Bodies, Saving Souls: A History of Hospitals*. New York: Oxford University Press, 1999.

Rosenberg, Charles. *The Care of Strangers: The Rise of America's Hospital System*. Baltimore: Johns Hopkins University Press, 1987.

Rosenfield, Isadore, and Zachary Rosenfield. *Hospital Architecture and Beyond*. New York: Van Nostrand Reinhold, 1969.

Seiter, Ellen. *Television and New Media Audiences*. New York: Oxford University Press, 1999.

Serlin, David, ed. *Imagining Illness: Public Health and Visual Culture*. Minneapolis: University of Minnesota Press, 2010.

———. "Performing Live Surgery on Television and the Internet since 1945." In *Imagining Illness: Public Health and Visual Culture*, edited by David Serlin, 223–44. Minneapolis: University of Minnesota Press, 2010.

Shattuc, Jane. *The Talking Cure: TV Talk Shows and Women*. New York: Routledge, 1997.

Singer, Ben. *Melodrama and Modernity*. New York: Columbia University Press, 2001.

Slide, Anthony. *Before Video: A History of the Non-theatrical Film*. New York: Greenwood Press, 1992.

Spigel, Lynn. *Make Room for TV: Television and the Family Ideal in Postwar America*. Chicago: University of Chicago Press, 1992.

Stacey, Jackie. *Teratologies: A Cultural Study of Cancer.* London: Routledge, 1997.
Staiger, Janet. *Interpreting Films: Studies in the Historical Reception of American Cinema.* Princeton: Princeton University Press, 1992.
Starr, Paul. *The Social Transformation of American Medicine: The Rise of a Sovereign Profession and the Making of a Vast Industry.* New York: Basic, 1984.
Sternberg, Esther M. *Healing Spaces: The Science of Place and Well-Being.* Cambridge: Harvard University Press, 2009.
Sterne, Jonathan. *The Audible Past: Cultural Origins of Sound Reproduction.* Durham: Duke University Press, 2003.
Stevens, Rosemary. *In Sickness and in Wealth: American Hospitals in the Twentieth Century.* Baltimore: Johns Hopkins University Press, 1999.
Stevens, Rosemary, Charles E. Rosenberg, and Lawton R. Burns, eds. *History and Health Policy in the United States: Putting the Past Back In.* New Brunswick: Rutgers University Press, 2006.
Terry, Jennifer, and Melodie Calvert, eds. *Processed Lives: Gender and Technology in Everyday Life.* New York: Routledge, 1997.
Thompson, John D., and Grace Goldin. *The Hospital: A Social and Architectural History.* New Haven: Yale University Press, 1975.
Thompson, Robert. *Television's Second Golden Age: From* Hill Street Blues *to* ER. Syracuse: Syracuse University Press, 1997.
Tiefer, Leonore. "The Medicalization of Impotence: Normalizing Phallocentrism." *Gender Society* 8, no. 3 (1994): 363–77.
———. *Sex Is Not a Natural Act, and Other Essays.* Boulder: Westview, 1995.
———. "The Viagra Phenomenon." *Sexualities* 9, no. 3 (2006): 275.
Tomes, Nancy. "Patients or Health-Care Consumers? Why the History of Contested Terms Matters." In *History and Health Policy in the United States: Putting the Past Back In*, edited by Rosemary Stevens, Charles E. Rosenberg, and Lawton R. Burns, 83–110. New Brunswick: Rutgers University Press, 2006.
Torrey, E. Fuller. *Out of the Shadows: Confronting America's Mental Illness Crisis.* New York: Wiley, 1998.
Treichler, Paula. *How to Have Theory in an Epidemic.* Durham: Duke University Press, 1999.
Treichler, Paula, Lisa Cartwright, and Constance Penley, eds. *The Visible Woman: Imaging Technologies, Gender, and Science.* New York: New York University Press, 1998.
Turow, Joseph. *Playing Doctor: Television, Storytelling, and Medical Power.* New York: Oxford University Press, 1989.
Ulrich, Roger. "Biophilic Theory and Research for Healthcare Design." In *Biophilic Design: The Theory, Science and Practice of Bringing Buildings to Life*, edited by Stephen R. Kellert, Judith Heerwagen, and Martin Mador, 87–106. Hoboken: Wiley.

———. "Effects of Health Facility Interior Design on Wellness: Theory and Recent Scientific Research." *Journal of Healthcare Design* 3 (1991): 99.
———. "A Theory of Supportive Design for Healthcare Facilities." *Journal of Healthcare Design* 9 (1997): 3–7.
———. "View through a Window May Influence Recovery from Surgery." *Science* 224, no. 4647 (1984): 420–21.
Upton, Dell. *Architecture in the United States*. Oxford: Oxford University Press, 1998.
Vares, Tiina, and Virginia Braun. "Spreading the Word, but What Word Is That? Viagra and Male Sexuality in Popular Culture." *Sexualities* 9, no. 3 (2006): 315–32.
Verderber, Stephen, and David J. Fine. *Health Care Architecture in an Era of Radical Transformation*. New Haven: Yale University Press, 2000.
Verderber, Stephen, and David Reuman. "Windows, Views, and Health Status in Hospital Therapeutic Environments." *Journal of Architectural Planning and Research* 4, no. 1 (1987): 121–33.
Waldby, Cathy. *AIDS and the Body Politic: Biomedicine and Sexual Difference*. London: Routledge, 1996.
Watkins, Elizabeth. *On the Pill: A Social History of Oral Contraceptives, 1950–1970*. Baltimore: Johns Hopkins University Press, 1998.
Watney, Simon. *Policing Desire: Pornography, AIDS, and the Media*. 2nd ed. Minneapolis: University of Minnesota Press, 1997.
Weber, Brenda R. *Makeover TV: Selfhood, Citizenship, and Celebrity*. Durham: Duke University Press, 2009.
White, Michele. *The Body and the Screen: Theories of Internet Spectatorship*. Cambridge: MIT Press, 2006.
White, Mimi. *Tele-advising: Therapeutic Discourse in American Television*. Chapel Hill: University of North Carolina Press, 1992.
Wildman, Rachel P., Paul Muntner, Kristi Reynolds, Aileen P. McGinn, Swapnil Rajpathak, Judith Wylie-Rosett, and MaryFran R. Sowers. "The Obese without Cardiometabolic Risk Factor Clustering and the Normal Weight with Cardiometabolic Risk Factor Clustering." *Archives of Internal Medicine* 168, no. 15 (2008): 1617–24.
Williams, Allison, ed. *Therapeutic Landscapes*. Surrey: Ashgate, 2008.
Williams, Raymond. *Keywords: A Vocabulary of Culture and Society*. New York: Oxford University Press, 1985.
———. *Television: Technology and Cultural Form*. Hanover: Wesleyan University Press, 1992.
Young, James Harvey. *The Medical Messiahs: A Social History of Health Quackery in Twentieth-Century America*. Princeton: Princeton University Press, 1992.
Zimmerman, Patricia. *Reel Families: A Social History of Amateur Film*. Bloomington: University of Indiana Press, 1995.

# Index

The letter *f* following a page number denotes a figure.

Adams, Annmarie, 54–55
advertisements: deinstitutionalization and, 75, 125; early, 24–25, 32–33; glorification of television in, 81–82; in *The Modern Hospital*, 32, 33, 43, 47, 51, 71, 74–75, 84, 87, 89; for radio, 24–26, 35, 41–47; spatial therapeutics and, 71, 72f, 74–75, 81–84, 85f, 86–87, 86f, 89, 92. *See also* drug advertising, prescription
aesthetics, therapeutic, 77
agency, conditional, 16, 101–3
American Medical Association (AMA), 173n11
Andaleeb, Syed Saad, 175n29
architecture. *See* spatial therapeutics
autonomy (of patient), therapeutic and economic, 16, 101–2. *See also* control, patient

"back at home," 84, 85f
Banet-Weiser, Sarah, 141
bankruptcies, medical, 172n3
biomedicalization, 14–15
Bourdieu, Pierre, 182n53
brand community, 133–34
brand-name awareness (prescription drugs), 110
Brinkley, John R., 41, 162n38
"broadcasting," 65–66
Burri, Regula Valerie, 140

Calasanti, Toni, 125–26
Charcot, Jean-Martin, 159n1
Chicago Silent Call Signal System, 45, 46f
children, visiting patients by television, 63, 64f
Civil Rights Act of 1964, 63
Clarke, Adele, 14
closed-circuit television (CCTV), 63, 64f, 87–89, 164n4
commercialism for the public good, 97–98
consumer choice, 101–2. *See also* control, patient

consumer model vs. patient model, 15–16, 17
consumer-patients, 3, 15–17; as quasi-consumers, 102; television as home remedy for, 91–92; turning patients/citizen-subjects into, 118
control, patient, 16, 60–62, 101–2; privatized listening and, 87, 88f
Cotrupi, Toni, 150

Deen, Paula, 1
deinstitutionalization of hospitals, 2, 67, 91, 150, 155n1; advertisements and, 75, 125; defined, 2, 155n1; entertainment media and, 32, 48; film and, 31; nature of, 13; patient-oriented media and, 81; radio and, 39, 48; spatial therapeutics and, 76; television and, 12, 56, 67, 73, 91, 94, 145
Dictograph Production Company, 47
direct-to-consumer (DTC) prescription drug advertising, 93–96; historical and economic context for, 97; as informative vs. manipulative, 98–107, 110; money spent on, 99, 113, 176n38; physicians and, 104–8; positioning the consumer-patient, 108–13
Discovery Communications, 142
Discovery Health Channel, 141–43
distraction, positive/therapeutic: film as, 23–24, 31; television as, 2, 60, 66–67, 73, 74, 83, 86f, 91, 145, 166n31
dramas, medical, 7, 147
drug advertising, prescription: market research and, 105–6; physicians and, 104–8. *See also* direct-to-consumer (DTC) prescription drug advertising
drug companies, as consumer-patient advocates, 108
drugs, naming of, 178n23

Dumit, Joseph, 140
Dyer, Richard, 1, 145

Eastman, George, 29, 161n15
Eastman Kodak Company, 32; Medical Division, 29, 32–35, 161nn15–16
empowerment. *See* control, patient
entertainment (private), therapeutic and economic value of, 62–66
Euclid-Glenville Hospital, 62–63

female patients, television as distraction for, 84, 86f
film (in hospitals), 23–25; connecting patients to outside world, 34, 34f; Hospital Happiness Movement and, 29–32; movies as medicine, 26–28; as therapeutic, 32–37
film spectatorship, 28–31, 35–37, 48, 161n20
First World War, patient entertainment during, 27, 145
Fisch, Henry, 132
Food and Drug Administration (FDA), 109–12, 173n10
Foucault, Michel, 127, 170n16
Friedman, Lester, 7

Geist, Patricia, 102
Gillespie, John A., 106–7
Gilman, Sander, 99–100
Grossberg, Lawrence, 55

Halberstam, Judith, 127–28
Harpo Productions, 141, 142
"Harry and Louise" advertising campaign, 101–2
Harvey, Paul, 115
healing, experience of, 43–44
Healium Network, 11
health care consumer, 15. *See also* consumer-patients
health care reform, 101–2, 158n32; Patient Protection and Affordable Care Act of 2010, 144, 150, 158n32

Health Insurance Association of America (HIAA), 101
health in the media, 7–8
Hill-Burton Act, 56
Hilmes, Michele, 39
HIV/AIDS and Viagra, 180n44
Hospital Happiness Movement, 29–32
*Hospital Management*, 40, 74–75, 82
hospital rooms, 58; humanizing through design, 57–60 (*see also* spatial therapeutics)
hospitals: humanizing through design, 56–60 (*see also* spatial therapeutics); medicalization, 170n16; urban, 63
Hospital Survey and Construction Act, 56

*I Love Lucy* (TV program), 93
interior design, 77–78. *See also* spatial therapeutics
intertextual humor in commercials, 116, 121, 122, 128–34, 136, 137, 179n30, 181n51
intertextuality, critical, 179n30

Jackson, Barbara Bund, 134

KFKB radio station, 41
King, Neal, 125–26
Kodascope projector, 32–34

Lammers, John C., 102
LeBlanc, Dudley J., 171n1
Lefebvre, Henri, 80–81
Letourneau, Charles, 66–67
Loe, Meika, 120, 127

magazines, 51, 52, 74–75, 78, 94. *See also Hospital Management*; *Modern Hospital, The*
Martin, Mark, 136
McCarthy, Anna, 8, 9, 148, 163n2
medicalization (of the modern home), 95, 96, 113, 151–52; adoption of telemedicine for home health care and, 172n4; biomedicalization and, 14–15; features of, 13–14; historical perspective on, 14; process of, 144; television and, 13, 50–51; Viagra and, 113, 116–19, 133–40, 144
medicine as a business, 103
mobile privatization, 66
*Modern Hospital, The*, 26, 29, 48, 52–53, 56, 57, 63–64; advertisements in, 32, 33, 43, 47, 51, 71, 74–75, 84, 87, 89
motion pictures. *See* film
Mullins, Shila Renee, 149
*Mutual Film Corporation v. Industrial Commission of Ohio*, 35, 36

NASCAR commercials, 109, 118, 128–33, 136
National Broadband Plan, 152
neoliberalism, 10, 14–15, 121–24, 133, 138
Neutra, Richard J., 57
Nightingale, Florence, 75–76
Noth, Paul, 104
nurse-call communication systems, 45, 46f, 47, 58, 89–90
nurses' labor, television as reducing, 67
nurses' station, 58

Obama, Barack, 158n32
Obama, Michelle, 184n19
Oprah Winfrey Network (OWN), 141

Palmeiro, Rafael, 131
patient/consumer, 15–17; contractions vs. expansions of powers of, 16. *See also* consumer-patients
Patient Protection and Affordable Care Act of 2010, 144, 150, 158n32
Pfizer, 103–4, 106–7. *See also* NASCAR commercials; Viagra

pharmaceutical companies, 108
pharmaceutical sales representatives (PSRs) and physicians, 175n29
Philco, 89, 90f
physicians: pharmaceutical sales representatives and, 175n29; prescription drug advertising and, 104–8; on television, 8
pillow speaker, 89
Potts, Annie, 124–25
Powerizer Sound Systems, 43
Presley, Elvis, 134–37
proximity of television to patient. *See* spatial therapeutics

racial differences in hospital accommodation, 65
radio, 37, 81; advertisements for, 24–26, 35, 41–47; contrasted with film, 37; early history, 23–24; as news of the well world, 37–48; and patient recovery, 41–42; prescribed to patients as therapeutic distraction, 31; public debates surrounding, 159n2; recuperative and privatized listening, 43, 44f
radio pillow, 165n47
Ray, Rachael, 1
reality television, 7, 143, 146–48, 183n16
relationship marketing and medicalization, 133–40
remote control devices, 45, 87–89, 90f
Rosenberg, Charles, 160n4

Seiter, Ellen, 5
self-determination. *See* control
sexuality, pharmaceuticals, and the neoliberal consumer-patient, 121–24, 133, 138. *See also* Viagra
sexuopharmaceuticals, 125. *See also* Viagra
silent signaling, 45, 46f
Simmons, Kelly, 130

*Simpsons, The* (TV program), 115–16
Smith, Mickey C., 105–6
Sollisch, Jim, 149
space, representations of, 80
spatial therapeutics, 71, 72f, 73, 119–20; advertisements and, 71, 72f, 74–75, 81–84, 85f, 86–87, 86f, 89, 92; definition and meanings of, 76, 120, 168n5; double-edged aspects of, 79; origin of the term, 6, 169n5; and the patient room, 75–79; process of, 144; of proximity, 79–91; of television, 6
Spigel, Lynn, 52, 58, 65–66, 160n5, 168n3
Stacey, Jackie, 175n32
Sterne, Jonathan, 39
Stevens, Rosemary, 51, 65
supportive design (hospital rooms), 59–60
Supreme Court, 35, 36

Tacconi, Leonard J., 143
Tallman, Robert F., 175n29
television (in the hospital): before, 97; integrated entertainment and therapeutic functions, 89, 90f; as machine for healing in megahospitals, 53–56; positioning (*see* spatial therapeutics); position of patient in relation to, 79–91; privatized listening and patient control, 87, 88f; as providing space to heal, 66–69; purposes, 2
television viewing, negative effects of, 68, 83
therapeutic discourse and television, 168–69n5
therapeutic landscape, 76
therapeutic positioning and repositioning, 9, 20, 73–75, 91, 96, 119–20, 139, 140. *See also* spatial therapeutics
therapeutic value, 4

Thomas, Marcus, 149
Thompson, Robert, 7
Tiefer, Leonore, 124–25
Tomes, Nancy, 15–17
Turow, Joseph, 7
Twiss, C. Victor, 78

Ulrich, Roger S., 59–62

Verderber, Stephen, 166n33
Viagra, 109; popular culture and, 115–17, 117f
Viagra brand, living within the, 133–40
Viagra studies and aging masculinity, 124–28
Viagra television commercials, 180n44, 180n46, 181nn51–52, 182n55; and the neoliberal consumer-patient, 121–24; sport and intertextual humor in, 116, 121, 128–34, 136, 137. *See also* Viva Viagra campaign

"video visits" with family and friends, 63, 64f
Viva Viagra campaign, 118, 133–37, 180n44

Wanamaker, Duane, 160n10
Watkins, Elizabeth, 124
Wazana, Ashley, 106
Weber, Brenda R., 10, 143
Western Electric, 43–45
Williams, Raymond, 12, 65, 66
windowness, 58
windows in hospital rooms, 58–59
Winfrey, Oprah, 141, 142, 169n5
women patients, television as distraction for, 84, 86f
World War I, patient entertainment during, 27, 145

Yates, Andrea, 174n20

Zenith, 87, 88f
Zoloft, 106–7

JOY V. FUQUA is assistant professor of media studies at Queens College, City University of New York.

Library of Congress Cataloging-in-Publication Data
Fuqua, Joy V., 1962–
Prescription TV : therapeutic discourse in the
hospital and at home / Joy V. Fuqua.
p. cm. Includes bibliographical references and index.
ISBN 978-0-8223-5115-3 (cloth : alk. paper)
ISBN 978-0-8223-5126-9 (pbk. : alk. paper)
1. Television broadcasting—Health aspects.
2. Television in medicine.
3. Hospital patients—Services for.
4. Patients—Services for.
I. Title.
PN1992.55.F87 2012
363.11′9792—dc23    2011053296

www.ingramcontent.com/pod-product-compliance
Lightning Source LLC
Chambersburg PA
CBHW051541230426
43669CB00015B/2680